A Twisted Fate

My Life With Dystonia

by Brenda Currey Lewis

Produced by:

FriesenPress

Suite 300 – 852 Fort Street
Victoria, BC, Canada V8W 1H8

www.friesenpress.com

Distributed to the trade by The Ingram Book Company

Preface

In the summer of 1974, at the age of seven, I started to experience odd, intermittent difficulties when walking. Soon I was walking on the outside of my foot all the time. Within a year, my right arm and leg were twisting and pulling to the extent that I required a rare form of brain surgery that held no promise of success. From then on my life was propelled down a bizarre roller coaster of ups and downs.

This book is about how I have lived my life thus far with a rare neurological movement disorder called dystonia. It is not a medical journal or a "How to Live Successfully With Dystonia" book, simply because that help doesn't exist. That is all up to the patient's symptoms and attitude. This is an account of my life before and after the onset of a life-altering disorder. It is how I remember things unfolding. Notes and documents saved by my mother helped a great deal. It is also a tribute to those who have helped make my life richer and more livable! I wrote this book to create awareness about dystonia. Its symptoms often make it difficult for doctors to diagnose. Some people with dystonia have been diagnosed by a friend or relative who stumbled upon a blurb in a newspaper or a news report. Perhaps my book will serve as a resource to help others get an early and correct diagnosis.

Symptoms come in a vast array of combinations that make each individual's condition unique. So I hope that I do each individual justice, knowing their symptoms are not exactly like mine.

Please consult a healthcare professional before taking any steps on my medical references alone!

Acknowledgements

First I would like to thank my computer; this book would not have been written without this technology! There were also many people who helped me, and I would like to thank them:

Dr. Wayne Martin, my neurologist at the Movement Disorder Clinic, who assisted me with medical terms and procedures.

Physiotherapists Chris Rodger and CariAnn Cooke, who assisted me with some terminology and anatomical references.

The Dystonia Medical Research Foundation and the Dystonia Medical Research Foundation Canada (DMRF-C) for providing quotes and explanations to better inform my readers.

Connie Zalmanowitz for keeping me up to speed on our fund-raising efforts and for all that she has done for the Edmonton Dystonia Support Group.

The Rick Hansen Foundation for allowing Mr. Hansen's story to be told, in part, through my story!

Brenda Currey Lewis

Special thanks to Dr. Ehor Gauk for his proficient diagnosis way back in 1974.

Dedication

To Mom, who was with me in most of my defining moments and kept notes and letters that helped make this book possible. To the rest of my family for their support and for making my life as interesting as it has been.

Mom has encouraged me over and over again to write my book. Among the letters she kept while I was hospitalized far from home, I came across one penned by my father on August 31, 1976. It said in part,

"Brenda you should write a book when all this is through. I am sure it will give strength to a lot of people who would have gone through a <u>lot</u> less than you have. God knows you're strong and only He knows how much stronger you'll be when it's all done."

Well, it isn't all done, but I feel it's the right time to tell 'my story.'

A Twisted Fate

Prologue

Parts of my body are starting to twist and move. Twisting, twisting, need to move, need to move, constant movement, and I don't know when it's going to stop. Something is totally out of control. My muscles are pulling and pushing against one another, long and hard enough to make my bones change and deform. Pull, pull, pull, wait it out. I have no other choice; breathe in and out and wait it out. I want to reach that chair not more than ten feet away. Okay, Brenda, I tell myself, put one foot firmly on the ground, heel first, then the next and repeat — the way you've always done it. "Sorry," my muscles say, "but that's not going to happen". My right foot arches and turns onto its outer edge. This seems to be my only option. Why? I take the step anyway and am thrown off balance. Sometimes I fall. Other times, looking awkward, I manage to right myself especially if there is something secure that I can grab onto. What is my pelvis doing? Somehow it's protruding forward, throwing me off balance. Why can't I stop it? I'm not asking for this. Hey, what's with my right arm? My hand is cramping and clenching while my arm is pulling behind my body. I should be able to stop this. A few months ago, I wasn't doing any of this. When I sit, my right leg pulls up toward my chest at an odd angle. That's funny; it feels good and natural! How can that be? But I must try to sit normally— this is embarrassing! For a second or two I can sit fine and then the muscles insist on going back to the weird posturing. What's going on? Pretty bizarre things are happening. I don't understand, I'm seven years old. I haven't seen anyone else doing this. What's happening? What am I doing wrong?

Introduction

DYSTONIA is a neurological movement disorder that causes muscles to contract and spasm involuntarily. The neurological mechanism that makes muscles relax when they are not in use does not function properly. Opposing muscles often contract simultaneously as if they are 'competing' for control of a body part. The involuntary muscle contractions force the body into repetitive and often twisting movements as well as awkward, irregular postures. Dystonia is the third most common movement disorder next only to Parkinson's Disease and Tremor. While it is a chronic disorder, the overwhelming majority of cases are not fatal. Estimates suggest that no fewer than 300, 000 people in North America are affected. But that is just the tip of the iceberg when it comes to understanding the true prevalence of all types of dystonias.

Brenda Currey Lewis

(Courtesy of the Dystonia Medical
Research Foundation Canada)

There are approximately thirteen types of dystonia. The type I have is called dystonia musculorum deformans or generalized dystonia for short. All the other types are described at the end of this book. Everyone's experience with dystonia is different. There's no measuring stick for people with physical problems. Symptoms, and their severity, vary among people with dystonia. It takes an average of seven years for a correct diagnosis. Various treatments work well to moderate for some people but are ineffective for others. There seems to be an exception to every rule. Everyone has a story. This is *my story*.

Dystonia has been an unwelcome companion since 1974. My torso is twisted and my left hip continually straightens and twists inward; therefore, my left leg refuses to stay on the foot pedal of my wheelchair. My leg demands to stick out to the side, whether I'm sitting or standing, and ultimately gets its way. My left knee needs to straighten too, and my foot clenches quite vigorously most of the time. Many medications, surgeries, and failed interventions have taken place over the years. My right side has been rescued from the tyrant that invaded it, but my left shoulder and arm have a permanent tremor.

It's been a long battle to get me to where I am today. Most people who verbalize their thoughts to me ask if I have multiple sclerosis or have had an accident of some kind. When I tell them I have a rare neurological disorder called dystonia, they usually draw a blank. That needs to change.

The lack of awareness about dystonia motivated me to write this book. I hope my story will interest and educate you, expand your beliefs and attitudes about people with differences, make you laugh and maybe even cry. But the main objective is to spread the word about dystonia: what it is, how it affects people, and why more research is needed to find better treatments and eventually a cure for this unwelcome intruder. Although some forms are hereditary, some cases show up with no family history. Dystonia can happen to anyone!

This is about my life dealing with dystonia and all the other ups and downs that came my way. I hope I do justice for all who have this disease. Every case is different yet so much the same! I was living a life that took a drastic turn at a young age. I had to face it. I had no choice. This is how it's gone!

Chapter 1

March 20, 1967 started out like any other day of my mother's third and last pregnancy. It was her due date, so she hoped that things would be different. She anticipated feeling contractions and her water breaking. She went to see her doctor, but all he could do was tell her to go home and drink some cod liver oil. That did the trick. She awoke at midnight, and less than an hour and a half later I was born to loving parents Sheron and Richard Currey. It was a normal, routine delivery. I had all ten fingers and toes, and everything was where it should have been.

My birthday, March 21, was the first day of Spring and I was the first—and only—child to inherit my mom's red hair. I have two siblings; Kevin was born in 1962, and Trisha was born in 1963. We had no idea that I had also inherited an unwanted recessive gene.

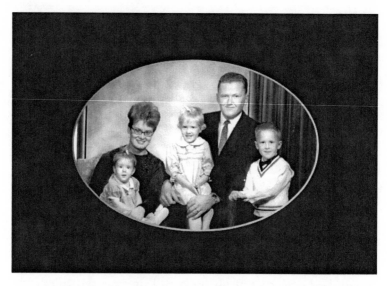

My family. Me, Mom, Trisha, Dad and Kevin in 1967

My life got off to a good start. I was a typical pre-schooler—inquisitive and active. My earliest memories are of bedtime. My sister and I shared a room in our three-bedroom bungalow until my parents could construct a bedroom in the basement for my brother. As the younger sister, I usually went to bed earlier than Trisha did. When I got into bed I would cover myself and pretend I wasn't there, and my mom would pretend she didn't know where I was. She would search my room for a minute and then pull back the covers. I loved to see the look of surprise on her face when she found me under the covers. My parents raised me with a lot of love and security—and a little more discipline than I would have liked-—but that has helped mold the person I have become.

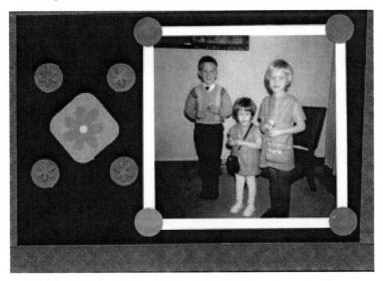

We're all dressed up in 1969

Mom enrolled me in piano lessons when I was six years old. I didn't like it too much, but I made it through two grades. I loved getting stickers for improving my skills, so I gave it my best shot. Attending school was what I really looked forward to. I was quite excited when I started grade one. Every day I rushed home to read to my mom from the standard issue 'See Spot Run' books. Sometimes I would stay after class and help my teacher, Mrs. Campbell, clean up, so Mom would have to come looking for me.

I was the tallest student in my grade one class. When our school gave out little spruce trees for every first grader to take home and plant in their yard, I was last in line because of my height. The trees were well picked over, and the few I had to pick from were pretty spindly. Because of my height, I was a bit less graceful than others—I could never quite clear a hurdle during sports day, and I wasn't crazy about gym class—but I was just as active as any other child I knew.

I remember my first bicycle. It was blue and had a white banana seat with brightly coloured flowers all over it. It was very typical in the early 1970s. I loved riding it very much. Once I was riding it down our driveway, unaware that a car was coming down the lane. The moment before the car would have hit me I braked so fast I fell sideways into a patch of stinkweed. The stinkweed was teeming with miniature spiders! This did nothing to decrease my dislike and fear of insects.

Mom and Dad made a great effort to take us on a family vacation every summer. For three summers in a row we drove through the Rocky Mountains of Alberta and British Columbia to go to Shuswap Lake. It was a long twelve hours, especially in the summer heat with no air conditioning and so little room for us three kids in the back seat. No one wanted the dreaded middle seat. It was quite an adventure driving through and beside mountains and stopping at hot springs along the way.

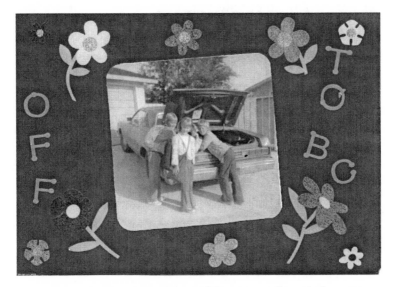

Leaving for Shuswap Lake. Trisha, me, and Kevin in 1973

And when we got to the Shuswap it was heaven! We stayed at a great little community of rented pine cabins. We walked to the main cabin to sign out canoes, paddle boats, shuffle board and ping pong equipment. The owners of the cabin community had a boat and would take anyone water skiing. My brother picked up that skill very quickly. The pier was intimidating because of the gap between its sections. This gap was not huge, but it could have been the opening to Mount St. Helens for all I knew. I had to drum up the courage every time to make the small leap to the next section of the dock.

I loved the water, although I could not swim. I liked the inner tubes and air mattresses. Fellow vacationers encouraged me to put my head under the water. I found it hard to work up the courage to do it. Finally one friendly lady said she would give me a dime if I would dunk my head. A dime would definitely buy me a treat, but I still needed a lot of coaxing before I took the plunge. And I even lived to tell about it!

There was a wonderful sandy beach where all us kids made big sand castles. At the same beach, fellow campers gathered for a bonfire and roasted hotdogs and marsh-mallows as the mid – summer sun went down. Some older kids would tell scary ghost stories. After that, I was always hesitant to walk outside when the sun went down.

Every so often Kevin, Trisha and I got some spend-ing money, so we'd walk down the hot gravel road to the candy store. I loved sponge toffee first and foremost, and it was the first thing I bought with the dime I earned from dunking my head. We found it amusing when two young boys entered the store exclaiming that they could buy everything in the store with the money they had acquired. It was Monopoly money!

The hot summers were a welcome contrast to our cold, snowy prairie winters. But we stayed active in the winter time too. My parents introduced me to snow skiing when I was about five years of age. At Snow Valley, a ski hill in Edmonton, I used a tow rope or a T-bar to get to the top of the hill. On my way down the hill there was a mogul I anticipated and feared so much that I fell before I got to it every time. We also skied in the Rocky Mountains and rode the chair lifts. But I was never one for just playing outside at home. My mom would often dress me up in my snowsuit and stick me outside in the backyard for some fresh air. I would get so cold and bored I would sit by the door and occasionally ring the doorbell until she would let me back in.

Christmas was always a magical time of year for me—the sparkles, colours, hymns, and food—and playing an angel in the church pageant was always something I looked forward to. The Christmas of 1973, I unwrapped a pair of brand new white ice skates. I was so excited. One day soon after, Dad,—who as a long-time hockey referee was no stranger to skating rinks—took the three of us to the Jasper Place skating rink, a few blocks from our home. The moment my blades touched the ice I felt unstable. That is fairly normal for a first time on skates, but try as I might I could not even stand still on my own. My right foot kept turning inward as though my ankle was weak, but under normal circumstances it was fine. Practice was making things worse instead of better. Dad got upset because I would not skate or even stand on my own; I kept gripping his leg. I was mystified and frustrated by what was taking place. After a while our fun afternoon at the rink was cut short, and we all walked home in silence.

The frustration I experienced at the skating rink was unusual for me; according to my mom, I was an extremely patient child. While learning to tie my shoes, I diligently started over and over again until I finally got it right. I was patient even when I was playing with my sister. We had a space in the basement, under the stairs, that we made into a small play area. My sister pretended she was a dental hygienist and asked me to sit in the waiting room while she prepared the small space for my appointment. She had a small cup of lemon juice she used as fluoride and applied it to my teeth with a Q-tip. Mom had worked for a dentist in earlier days and had brought home one of those tiny mirrors that they stick in a patient's mouth to see places otherwise not visible to them. The waiting room was a small section in the laundry room. Mom would come and go and see me waiting patiently. Trisha left me sitting in her waiting room for prolonged periods of time. Apparently I didn't mind waiting because I liked playing with my sister. I wanted her approval, so I waited. The sitting and waiting for appointments certainly fore-shadowed events of the years to come!

Chapter 2

In 1974, within three months after my 7th birthday, major changes started happening. I walked around in bare feet most of the time while we were at a local campground on a summer long weekend. Mom and Dad strongly sensed that something was wrong. I had started to drag my right foot and put weight on the outside of it in response to a strange tugging sensation. Mom touched and gently slapped my lower leg and foot to see if there was pain or numbness. When she asked why I was walking that way, I could not answer that question. *Why would it be preferable to stand and walk on the edge of my foot instead of flat-footed like everyone else?* There was nothing to be gained by walking that way. My walking had started to get very awkward, but I honestly didn't know why.

After seeing our family doctor, we were none the wiser. She sensed something was seriously wrong, so she referred us to a neurologist. I had to miss the first day of grade two in order to see this doctor. The neurologist examined me thoroughly. He did an electromyography

(EMG) which detects the electrical potential generated by muscle cells when these cells are mechanically active or at rest. He also did an electroencephalography (EEG) which records brain activity and is used to detect epilepsy, tumours, strokes and brain death. (These tests have generally been replaced by magnetic resonance imaging (MRI) and computerized axial tomography (CAT) scans).

Peripheral nerve damage in my knee was his diagnosis. He sent me to an orthopedic doctor who wrapped my knee in gauze and sent me home. When the gauze proved useless, which didn't take long, he put me in a fiberglass walking cast. That didn't work either. Next he fitted me with a heavy metal brace to keep my right foot in the proper position in my shoe when I walked. If anything, this aggravated the problem and increased my frustration level.

My muscles rebelled, but I had to wear the brace and orthopedic shoes anyway. When I was in grade one I had a favorite pair of shoes. They were brown and had a low square heel. I felt so grown up when I was wearing them. Instead, I had to wear orthopedic shoes that were ugly and embarrassing. They were hard leather and more difficult to put on than any other shoe I had worn. To walk I had to drag my right foot behind me while my muscles were throwing me off balance.

Shortly after my foot started to give me problems, Mom noticed I was doing activities such as eating and brushing my teeth with my left hand. I had always been right-handed. Back to the doctor's office we went. Since this neurologist hadn't a clue what was wrong, he told my mom that I was simply seeking attention!

Mom demanded a second opinion because she knew me better than that. She now started to wonder about Rob, a distant relative in my father's family, who had a rare brain disease. Nobody knew much about it; it was never talked about. We had another relative, Dr. Les Dushinski, who at that time was a urologist at the Royal Alexandra Hospital, commonly known as the Royal Alex. He knew a fellow doctor, Dr. Gauk, very well. He was the pediatric neurologist practicing at the Royal Alex. The November of my second year at school, I had my first appointment. With Dr. Dushinski's help we were able to get into see him within two months. Chances are, had we not known Dr. Dushinski, we would have had to wait much longer.

Dr. Gauk's office was on the main floor of the Children's Pavilion of the Royal Alexandra, right next to the elevator. Little Bo Peep characters adorned the elevator walls. After a short examination, he decided to admit me to the hospital so he could get to the bottom of my problem. They found me a bed in the Children's Pavilion. We liked Dr. Gauk very much. He quickly gained our trust through his sincerity and incredibly comforting bedside manner. He truly had found his calling.

I was hospitalized for two weeks. I recalled visiting my dad a couple of years earlier when he had surgery for a hernia. Hospital rules dictated that we stay in the main lobby while he came down in a wheelchair to visit us. But this was the first time I had ever been a patient.

The children's ward was vibrant and busy. More beloved fairy tale characters adorned all the internal windows of the ward. I had to eat in the playroom with all the other kids unless I was too sick. Being quite shy when it came to strangers, I would have preferred to eat in my room. I got many cute cards, flowers and little gifts from various friends and relatives. One card had ten dimes taped to the inside so I would be able to use the payphone, the only way to call home. Because I instantaneously liked Dr. Gauk, I looked forward to doctor's rounds. Dr. Gauk would come through the door in his short lab coat with a black bag full of medical instruments and tagging along behind him, a group of interns or residents.

A pneumoencephalography (PEG) was the last of an array of tests that he ordered. During this test, a small amount of cerebral spinal fluid is drained and replaced with air, oxygen, or helium so that x-rays of the brain show up more clearly. This procedure was fairly dangerous and caused severe headaches and vomiting over a long recovery period. I learned that the hard way! By the late 1980s this test was largely abandoned in favor of emerging MRI technology.

In preparation for this invasive procedure, I was lightly sedated before I left the ward. The test was scheduled so early in the morning that the ward was darker and quieter than usual. For two full weeks prior they had done every basic test, including x-rays and an E.E.G. to monitor my brain's activity. None of the test results showed any problems.

The stretcher arrived and we crossed the windowed pedway to the main hospital. I remember being lifted from the stretcher and set onto a chair. This chair was so comfortable it was like they had it tailor-made just for me and my size. It was lined with sheepskin, or something similarly soft. I was so comfy I felt like I was on a cloud. I recently found out this was a special chair designed for this procedure that enabled the patient's head to get as close as possible to the equipment involved. It seems funny to me that I have always remembered that chair! The light sedation earlier made it possible to relax and enjoy the fleeting moments until I was asleep. They reclined the chair so that my head, neck, and spine were most accessible to the table and equipment. Then it was lights out for me for the next hour or so. They removed the fluid from around my brain and pumped air into my brain tissue. Upon waking I was instantly aware of a terrible headache that lasted for days. I guess when you have air sent up to your brain, that's what's going to happen. After this test I could no longer tolerate headaches, even the mildest of them. The only consolation to having this test at a young age was that I was put to sleep. If I were an adult, I would have had to be awake for this procedure. More foreshadowing!

I went home a few days later in my mom's 1970 Toyota Corolla. She reclined the passenger seat, but it was little help. I still felt nauseated by every bump or pothole we drove over. As much as I wanted to get home, I asked her to slow down!

Chapter 3

Shortly before that agonizing ride home, Mom and Dad had been ushered into Dr. Gauk's office. My Grandma and my mom's three sisters, who had all come along for moral support, sat patiently in the waiting room while Dr. Gauk gave my parents his diagnosis.

It was dystonia musculorum deformans or generalized dystonia for short. I was a textbook case: between the age of five and fourteen years, lower limb turning inward forcing me to walk on the outer edge of my foot, and the disease was progressing upward.

Years later Dr. Gauk said he knew right off the bat what was wrong. If it looked like a duck, quacked like a duck, and swam like a duck, it was probably a duck, but he had to rule out all other possibilities first. We were grateful that my doctor had seen a few cases before, because the only way to be diagnosed is to find a doctor who recognizes the outward movements and twisting motions. He had only seen a few cases in Edmonton and other cities he had practiced in. Ironically one had been the distant relative, Rob, whom my mom had wondered about. This condition is hereditary in my case. My mom told Dr. Gauk that she didn't know whether to laugh or cry, because she did not know what life with dystonia musculorum deformans would mean for me. Dr. Gauk answered that she could laugh because it wasn't a tumour and it wasn't deadly. The muscles themselves have nothing wrong with them, but opposing muscles compete. Messages sent from my brain to my muscles were working overtime. It is most likely caused by a chemical imbalance—over-stimulation from excess chemicals—but little is known about how it manifests itself in the brain. They do know it is chronic with no cure or guaranteed effective treatment available. Nor is there any way to predict where or when it will end. What body parts will be affected? What intensity will these muscle spasms take on? The road ahead of us was going to be a long one!

Chapter 4

I had now entered the sterile and far-reaching world of doctor's waiting rooms, exam rooms, operating rooms, prosthetics departments, seating clinics, physical and occupational therapy, hospitals, new schools and transportation issues. In our wildest dreams we could not have imagined the magnitude of this new reality. There was now a hard core meaning to the word 'waiting.' It was no longer pretend, superficial waiting during play time. At times the physical and emotional strain caused by having to wait so much bordered on excruciating.

Mom asked Dr. Gauk what was to happen next. His advice was to do nothing for the moment. Watch and see if or how it progressed, because each case is different. They tried several different medications, but nothing seemed to make a significant difference. My mom had heard that Rob had surgery that was successful, and naturally she wanted the same for me. The story I heard at the time was that he entered the hospital needing a wheelchair, and after brain surgery he left the hospital walking independently. At that time Mom didn't know how serious and delicate the brain surgery, a thalamotomy, was. But she thought I deserved it and should have that opportunity.

Coincidentally, the evening after my diagnosis, grandma had been watching the TV medial drama, "Marcus Welby, MD." That evening's episode, *Hell's Upstairs*, was about a child with dystonia! That's what she had just been told her granddaughter had. She called my mom to let her know, but Mom was not in the right frame of mind to watch it. At the end of that episode a doctor's name was put up on the screen. Dr. Irving Cooper, who worked at St. Barnabas Hospital in New York City, performed that particular type of brain surgery. Eventually Dr. Gauk booked us an appointment with this surgeon, but upon further investigation he found a doctor in Toronto who was qualified and willing to do the thalamotomy on a child. At my time of need, there was not a doctor in Edmonton who would do this surgery on an eight year old. We could stay in Canada to get what I needed which made everyone feel more at ease. My mom was eager to see him immediately. Well, it didn't happen immediately, so in the meantime we carried on as best as we could.

Grade two was a year of drastic change for me and my family. We didn't live far from Meadowlark Public School, but now I was being driven the short distance.

My grade one class had been on the main floor, but my grade two class was regrettably on the second floor. At first I pulled myself up the stairs and, using the hallway coat racks for stability, walked awkwardly, and dragged my heavily-braced foot to my classroom. Mom consulted with my teacher, Mrs. Kelso, about having a throw rug where I could lie down when I got tired. I was like any other child, not wanting to be different or to stick out in the crowd, so I avoided using it.

Any friends I had from the previous year were in the other grade two class. One of those friends, a neighbor whose mom used to babysit me, started avoiding me when my symptoms developed. It bothered me, and I didn't understand her actions.

Fortunately, some people were accepting and helpful. It didn't take long to discover what a wonderful teacher Mrs. Kelso was. She was from Australia. She was very nice and accommodating. During recess I could not go outside anymore, and I remember sitting in the classroom and waiting for those very long fifteen minutes to end. A friend in the third grade quite often stood in the doorway to keep me company. He was not allowed to actually come in the room, but I still enjoyed his company from the doorway.

The previous year, my siblings and I walked home for lunch, but I now had to bring a bagged lunch along. The lunch room was downstairs — another obstacle for me.

Eventually two adults resorted to intertwining their arms to make a seat to get me to the lunch room. I didn't want that kind of attention, but I could not get there on my own steam. The time came in grade two when not only was I driven to school, I was also carried up and down the school stairwell every day. I was absolutely mortified by this kind of attention, and this was only the beginning!

People's perceptions change when they see an individual who has anything more than a simple limp. It seemed to me that intelligence, hearing, and other abilities are also questioned. So right from the get – go, in 1974 how I related to others, especially those my own age, and how they related to me, started to change. I wasn't living their lives, and they were not living mine. I noticed soon after my physical problems presented themselves that I was being treated differently than the able – bodied people around me. People telling me what I could and could not do was the main issue. But once I was aware of it, I felt fiercely that I had something to prove! That was a sad state of affairs, although it's more of an equal playing field today.

The relative I referred to earlier, Rob, who has dystonia, is from my father's side of the family. The disorder is hereditary in our case — we're the only two with it that I know about — but it can still show up in people with no known family history. Rob is approximately fifteen years older than I am. Our first and only meeting, that

I remember, was at my Grandma and Grandpa Currey's 50th wedding anniversary in the summer of 1975. He appeared quite reserved, but we had a short conversation.

I hadn't had any contact with him since 1975, but I met up with him at a family function in 2012. He has an awkward gait and walks with a cane, but he does use a wheelchair under some circumstances. We talked and had very similar stories about how our journeys began. We were both young when our symptoms began, first in a foot, and the hand and arm symptoms started not long after. His focus these days is on pain management. I had little contact with anyone going through the same thing I was. I will admit that it used to make me very nervous and uncomfortable to be around others with my disorder. It was an irrational fear, but perhaps I thought that their symptoms would rub off on me!

Fortunately I don't have any other relatives who have been diagnosed with dystonia, and the odds are very low that I will, but I hope that now I could be of assistance to whomever may become afflicted with it.

Chapter 5

Being diagnosed with dystonia musculorum deformans was, to say the least, confusing and frustrating. But being seven years old, I wasn't thinking down the line. I was just having to deal with the now. Believe me, the nights I couldn't get to sleep the question "Why?" raced through my head. What have I done? Am I a bad person? Did I harm anyone? I would think of silly things like, hadn't I done something that I had been asked to do, hadn't I cleaned my room like I was told? *WHAT?*

You can probably imagine that sleeping was a problem. Dystonia doesn't shut down just because you want it to or because you are ready to go to sleep. Many nights I would lie for hours in discomfort. By 2:00 or 3:00 in the morning I would debate whether I should wake my mom for her comforting advice and loving words or let her sleep. I didn't want to wake her, but I was at a loss as to what to do. Our house was fairly small and our bedrooms were close together. Every so often I would cry and she would hear me, although I tried hard not to let that happen. Those were the times when mom professed that she or my dad would do anything they could to take this burden on themselves so I would not have to suffer. I do wish that losing this burden was possible, but I wouldn't want anyone I love to go through this. When I'd finally get to sleep, my movements would cease. Mom and Dad would often open my door when they went to bed just to see my body and mind lying still and peaceful.

Once the diagnosis was made, the disease progressed very quickly. My right arm and leg were held captive by their own muscles, not free to move in the normal way. My arm was twisted and pulled behind me. My hand was a solid clenched fist. When I sat down, my right leg drew up tightly to my chest at an awkward angle. When I stood, that leg pulled back behind me making walking extremely awkward and laboured. My pelvis had a mind of its own. My mom and dad's approach to helping me stand straight was to rein in my protruding pelvis. They meant well, and their logic was sound for people with normal muscle control, but my pelvis fought back, working against them and me. My right foot teetered on its outside edge and arched so much I could not keep my heel in my shoe. My right leg crossed behind my left leg, and my right arm and clenched fist were thrust behind me. I would be frustrated in a terrible way. No one really understood. Especially me! What was happening? And why?

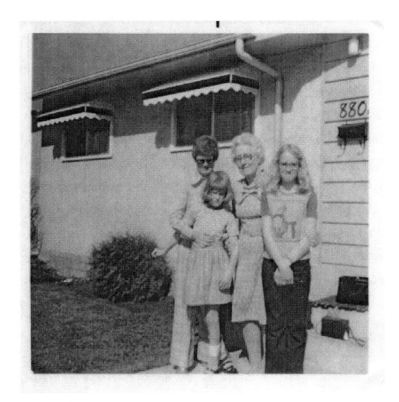

Not a happy camper! Mom trying to hold in my pelvis while my right leg and arm are pulling and twisted behind me. Standing with Mom, Great Aunt Stella and Trisha in 1975.

I had started taking medications that were designed, for the most part, to relax muscles. Over the years I've tried many different drugs but haven't found one that brings positive, long-lasting results. I can't say with any certainty that the drugs help at all. I have good days and bad days, so I've never known what to take away from that. The list of medications I've tried is very long, but some of the more common drugs include Baclofen, Benzatropine and Artane. All these drugs come with side effects.

Medications are effective for some people with dystonia. I have a friend, Janice, whose doctor managed to find the right combination of medication that brought such miraculous results she was able to finish university and go on to be a teacher. She says that she is somewhat of a medical mystery because these drugs have been keeping her dystonia in check for years, which is extremely rare. Her movements were severe before her doctor found the right combination of medications. She still has unwanted movement but it has slowed down by a big margin. This is another example of how individualized this disorder is. The type and severity of symptoms experienced and their responses to treatment vary from person to person.

Since the medications that Dr. Gauk had hoped would help were not making much of a difference, he thought the best thing for me now was to have the brain surgery, a thalamotomy. This was the surgery my mother had heard about. It was also the surgery that had been featured on the "Marcus Welby, M.D." episode. Rob had this particular surgery years earlier and it was very successful, for a time anyway. His surgery was done years earlier in Edmonton. There were risks involved, but the possibility of success was there. There were no other options, so the wheels were put into motion. "Immediately" had turned into nearly six months, but on May 22, 1975 we headed to Toronto to see my new neurosurgeon, Dr. Tasker.

The trip was a big mystery. We had no idea what was going to happen. The moment the airplane door opened onto the Lester B. Pearson airport tarmac, a rush of late spring heat and humidity filled the air. This type of humidity was new to me. Edmonton has a much drier climate. We hoped it wasn't going to be like this for the duration of our, hopefully, short stay. I felt beads of sweat forming on my forehead within minutes. I was just going to have to get used to it.

Our initial outpatient appointment with Dr. Tasker was scheduled for the next day. My dad's arms were to be my legs until we got to the hospital to use one of their wheelchairs. It was too early to accept the reality that I should really have my own wheelchair. If the surgery was successful enough, I wouldn't need one. It turned out to be a few days until I was actually admitted, so Dad fought a battle of endurance. I was only eight years old and very thin, but my inability to control my muscles, combined with the hot, humid weather made touring downtown Toronto extremely taxing on my dad and his arms. But we were not going to stay in the hot hotel room day and night with this big bustling city to explore! We made the most of the time we had before being cooped up in a hospital ward.

The appointment with my neurosurgeon, Dr. Tasker went well despite the three – hour wait in the hot, humid, and stagnant air in the main foyer of the Toronto General Hospital. I don't remember much about the appointment, but I remember his office was very small and diagrams of the brain covered the walls. He was a very gentle man, about fifty years old, with a greying beard. He always explained things in detail, but in words we could understand.

He would perform the surgery in two stages. The first stage was a surgical procedure to prepare my brain for the thalamotomy which would take place approximately five days later. This involved putting me under general anesthesia, making an incision to access my brain, and then drilling a small hole at the top left side of my skull. The incision and the hole in my skull were not going to be very big, so they wouldn't have to shave much of my hair off at the front. (I don't recall all that was done during this procedure besides preparing and mapping my brain for the actual thalamotomy).

The second stage, the thalamotomy, was the most feared of the two-stage operation. Dr. Tasker explained that they would put me to sleep temporarily and then put my head in a vise that had three pin-like grips. One would hold onto the top of my head at my hair line, the others would stabilize the sides of my head. The vise was necessary to prohibit any head movement after a probe was inserted through the small hole previously drilled at the top left of my skull. This probe would be slowly and meticulously navigated through my grey matter until it reached the thalamus.

The thalamus serves as a relay station connecting the basil ganglia area of the brain with nerves that stimulate muscles to move. Dystonia is believed to originate in the basal ganglia area which is the centre for muscle coordination. The thalamus is not actually part of the basil ganglia, but it serves as a relay station connecting it to other areas of the brain. This whole area is deep within the brain, so reaching the thalamus was not an easy task.

After they threaded the probe through the thalamus, they would wake me up. At that point, Dr. Tasker explained, the probe would send a tingly, weird sensation through a specific group of muscles. I would have to tell them if the probe was stimulating the area we wanted it to. Once we located the specified area, they would cryogenically kill (freeze) the cells in the affected area. This was intended to kill overactive cells thought to be under dystonia's control and stop the involuntary movements.

I'm grateful that I had this surgery at a young age, because I may have let fear decide for me later on. My mom and dad had to decide for me, and Mom was always eager to try anything that might help. If one treatment was deemed unsuccessful, I could go back for more. I know that these decisions were excruciatingly difficult to make.

There was a two to five percent chance that complications such as hitting a blood vessel could occur. But they all agreed this was a small chance, and since we were there out of desperation the surgery was a go! Dr. Tasker made arrangements for me to be admitted on May 27th.

Chapter 6

Admitting day was so hot and humid! Fans were working overtime but not giving much relief. The waiting room was full of people fanning themselves with magazines trying to keep cool. Each desk had an admitting clerk clicking away on an early 70's electric typewriter. It seemed ironic that at eight years of age I was being admitted to the Toronto General Hospital when the Hospital for Sick Children was directly across the street. Dr. Tasker only operated in the Toronto General.

After I was admitted, my dad could not stay very long due to his responsibilities at home. He was anxious to see the results of the first, and hopefully last, thalamotomy, so he worked out a plan that allowed him to stay on for a few extra days. On one of those days he bumped into someone he knew in the hospital elevator. I did not remember Reverend Smith, but he had been our minister at Trinity United Church in Edmonton before he moved to Toronto a few years back. A friend from our church had contacted him about our situation. He came to visit and offered my mom a room in his family home for as long as she needed it. What a godsend. Although most of our expenses were covered by Alberta Blue Cross and Handicapped Children's Services, some were going to be out of pocket. Not only was a financial burden taken off her shoulders, she would have a family to come home to every night.

The Smiths had five children and a wonderful big old house that oozed character and history. They lived in one of those old neighborhoods that are lined with majestic trees providing plenty of shade and beauty. Toronto is a big city, and the Smith's did not live close to the hospital. Mom really got to know the subway system.

Unlike the ward I had been on back in Edmonton, this ward's walls and windows were not adorned with painted cartoon figures. The entire ward was monochromatic beige. The only splash of color—ranging from yellow, to pink, to blue—was on the bed sheets and a green Naugahyde chair in each room for visitors. Since I would be on an adult neurological unit, Mom and Dad thought it best if I were in a private room. They didn't know what I might be exposed to if I had adult roommates with severe neurological problems. I wouldn't always be in a private room when I was hospitalized, but I was for my first visit.

Hospital beds are not made for comfort. The sheets are thin and the blankets are not as soft and cuddly as they should be. They also have bars that go up at night so patients don't fall out of bed. On the nights I couldn't sleep because I couldn't find a position my whole body could agree on, I would occasionally find comfort in wedging myself between the bed and the cold, metal rails. They were close enough to the bed that I wouldn't slip through, yet far enough for me to squeeze between. I must have looked awkward, like I was playing a solo game of 'Twister' in order to find enough relief to fall asleep.

I went stir crazy inside those hospital walls during the week, and absolutely nothing happened during the weekend in the General. If I wasn't able to get out on the weekend, I don't know what I would have done. Fortunately on most weekends I got a one or two-day pass. We spent some weekends at the Smith's lovely old home. Their house was a great, relaxing place to be. The trees that lined the street must have been over a hundred years old. I remember going to one of Reverend Smith's church services. I would try to listen to the sermon, but I would get distracted by one thing or another. I remember whispering into my mom's ear, "Besides preaching on Sundays, what does he do the rest of the week?"

We also visited another family in Toronto. Dad was a salesman in the edible oil department of a meat packing plant. The head office was in Toronto, so my parents knew some people there through his work. There was one couple that my dad knew quite well. We visited them occasionally in their high-rise apartment. One day, this

retired couple drove us to Niagra Falls. The Falls were a
spectacular scene.

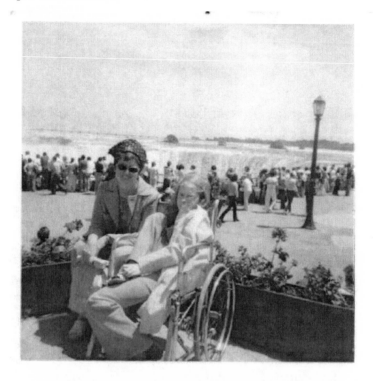

*Our day at Niagra Falls. The falls were beautiful, but I
was not able to sit normally or comfortably! 1975*

Some Saturdays we would just go walking down the
streets of downtown Toronto. The General Hospital was
centrally located, so we had easy access to some popular
areas. In the 1970s, downtown Toronto was more liberal
than Edmonton was. During one of our walks Mom considered taking a picture of me outside of a strip joint for
a laugh, but she quickly decided that probably wasn't all

A Twisted Fate

that funny or appropriate. So she took one of me outside
an arcade instead.

Chapter 7

The thought of brain surgery did not loom over me like a dark cloud. I took the news fairly well, but I was still scared. I was old enough to comprehend what was going to happen but too young to understand many of the details.

Two days after I was admitted, my preparatory surgery was done in an operating room that seemed very sterile, dark, and cold. I saw a masked doctor approach me with a big needle filled with neon green liquid. That was my personal take on the syringe's contents. At first I was intimidated by this big needle, but when I thought back to my spinal tap, during which I barely felt a thing while I was being anesthetized, I wasn't too worried. I had cause to worry. It was *the* most painful needle I've ever had! But I was out like a light in less than ten seconds. My mom explained afterward that the staff who anaesthetized me in Edmonton specialized in working with children. The staff at the Toronto General were not used to sticking huge needles into younger, more delicate body parts.

My first surgery was over. I spent some time in the recovery room and then went back to my room on the 10th floor. A simple, square Band – aid—the kind you can buy at your local drugstore—covered four stitches on my head.

I was scheduled to have the thalamotomy a few days later. This was the procedure that all our hopes rested upon. This one had the potential to do great things! Of course, anxiety before each surgery starts the night before, or even earlier, but what would finally make the surgery a complete reality, that I truly was going down-stairs for brain surgery any time now, was the preparation of my bed.

The nurses made the bed as usual while I watched from a chair. They unrolled a black canvas the length and width of a stretcher onto my bed. The canvas had six black ties sticking out, one on either side and two at each end. Then they covered the canvas with a blanket which I would lie on to await the orderly's impending arrival. That is when my heart started racing the fastest. The orderly would arrive way too soon with the stretcher, a metal frame designed to slide over top of me and under the bed simultaneously. He lowered it to bed level, threaded and fastened all six ties to the frame and raised it again to normal height. I felt like a picture in a frame! The wait for the elevator ended way too quickly. The worst scenario was having my surgery scheduled for the afternoon. The anxiety was bad enough, but on top of that, I couldn't eat or drink anything.

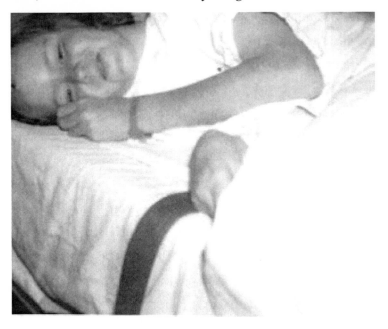

Waiting for surgery. Nervously smiling but anxiety ridden! Notice the black strap over the side of the bed?

The orderly took me to the surgical floor and left me on a stretcher next to the wall in the hallway. The floor was black with light speckles and the hallway lighting seemed dimmer than usual, but maybe that was because there were no windows on that floor. Hospital personnel ran around in their scrubs, complete with shoe covers, and colourful bandanas on their heads.

While I waited to be wheeled into the O.R., my trepidation escalated with every second that passed. The thing

I remember most while waiting—with my heart fluttering wildly in my chest—was being left next to a tiny, dimly lit room. Hanging in this space was a human spine. A nurse saw me staring at the spine in a terrified, yet curious way. She explained to me that this man had given his body to science after his death. I wondered if he ever imagined that his spine would be separated from the rest of his body and left hanging in a closet. I could only imagine where the rest of him went!

When the surgical team was ready, a nurse wheeled me into a different operating room than I was in a few days earlier. For the first time I entered the operating room where I would have all of my next eight surgeries. My first recollection was the door. It had a big vault-like knob. The room itself was on the small side and appeared much brighter than the O.R. I was in before. At the back of the room was a computer system panel. Back then it was high-tech; today it would seem primitive. I couldn't believe how much the room reminded me of a TV medical drama. There was the heart monitor screen, the pump that rose and fell, the big overhead lights, and lots of steel instruments. I don't how many medical shows were on the air at that time, but "Marcus Welby, MD" came to mind. Who else?

Having surgery would always make me vomit afterwards. The nausea was usually combined with a fever. That's all that this particular surgery produced! We were very hopeful, but there was no success. Dr. Tasker thought we should try again a few days later, so my father stayed in Toronto to see me through my second thalamotomy. He has always had sympathy for people—especially children—who suffer or have to endure procedures that few other people have to face. Because of his deep emotional state, my mom had two people to look after, not to mention herself. She really could only handle what I was going through. She would have loved to have him stay in Toronto every day for any support and company he could provide, but his emotional dependence limited his participation in that area and would have been much too hard to cope with. They knew Kevin and Trisha needed at least one parent at home to be there for them, and that could only be my dad.

After the second thalamotomy I actually got some relief. I could touch my right finger to my nose whereas previously my arm would not bend at all. I could stand properly with both feet flat foot on the floor and my leg could keep still. It felt great standing and moving my body fairly normally again! Things looked really good, and Dad went home with great news for everyone. Unfortunately the results didn't last long; later that day, as he was boarding the plane back to Edmonton, the movement started up again.

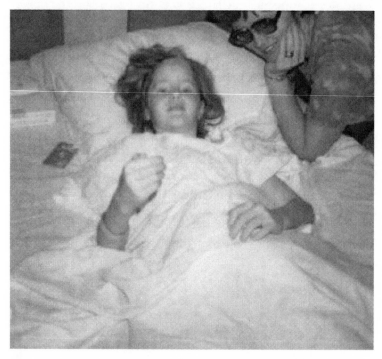

*Success! I could hold my arm up normally. My happy
mom is by my side. Success did not last long!*

Dr. Tasker was visibly upset and discouraged that the
good results had not lasted. He said he could do one more
if we wanted to try. We did, but it had no affect at all. We
went home to Edmonton soon after with deflated hearts.

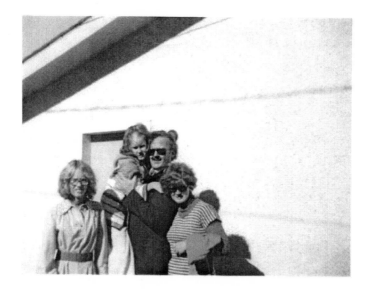

Just got home from Toronto in 1975 emotionally exhausted and disappointed. Trish, me secure in Dad's arms, and Mom.

Chapter 8

I was a quirky child. Whenever I cut myself or scraped my knee I would make quite a big production out of it. The only thing that could console me was getting a Band-aid on the wound. So after my first round of thalamotomies, a young nurse armed with a pair of scissors entered my room. The Band-aid had been taken off the incision on my skull a few days earlier, and this was the day my stitches were to come out. I wasn't sure if this was going to hurt, so I refused her request to take them out. She was frustrated because she told me it wouldn't hurt, but I didn't believe her. But I had a deep crush on a certain resident doctor, the one who removed my Band-aid. I believed that if he took my stitches out, it wouldn't hurt. So I said they could be taken out, but only by him, and that was my final compromise! So she went to find this doctor and he arrived a short time later. Having the stitches removed didn't really hurt, just a slight pulling sensation, so I was smiling with deep contentedness! I also wanted to keep the stitches as a memento, so the nurse found a small jar to put them in. I believe the jar and its contents did make it home, but somehow disappeared. My hunch was that my mom, not being as sentimental as I was, threw them away.

She may have thrown my stitches away, but while we were away from home my mom kept all the letters we received and even the ones we sent home. By doing so, she helped me document my journey, for the first few years anyway. At a time when email did not exist and long distance phone calls were tough on most people's budgets, we received many cards and letters. Notes from friends and family are priceless. People were great to me and didn't forget where I was or why. I got many get well cards, some with gifts or flowers. The correspondence between my mom and dad gives great insight into a young couple who loved each other and their children very much. My mom started her record keeping by writing "If I'd known this was going to be this long and involved, I would have started taking notes earlier...." When she heard that dystonia is probably a disorder based on a chemical imbalance, she automatically assumed and prayed that researchers would find a cure within a few years.

Between writing letters, and reading books, we killed some of the abundant time on our hands. During my first stay, Mom read *Pippy Longstocking* to me. My grade two classmates sent the book and letters from each of them.

I liked being read to and became an avid reader myself. Reading books such as *Charlie and the Chocolate Factory* made the hospital tutor's visits worthwhile. Doing school-work with the tutor was mandatory, but since I was in grade two, there wasn't much homework. I still love to read, but I don't do as much anymore because holding a book open at times, tends to make my body tense up.

Chapter 9

When we returned home after this first round of surgeries we were disappointed and emotionally exhausted. The surgeries left no lasting relief. It was obvious that I could no longer drag myself around, and my father could not always be there to carry me.

My condition got even worse than it was before we made the trip east. My *right* arm was sticking straight out behind me and would not allow me to bend it. I could only sit with my right leg bent up toward my chest at an outward angle. My lower back was starting to curve. The deforming part of dystonia musculorum deformans was now presenting itself. The time had come to use a wheelchair.

Every day when Dad came home from work he would change his clothes and then we would all sit down to a nice family dinner. But one day was very different. It was June 18th, 1975, the day after Mom and I returned home from Toronto. Dad came home and lugged a small, but bulky, wheelchair up the back steps. Seeing me sitting in my own wheelchair was heartbreaking for all of us, especially my parents. I remember the wheelchair feeling strange and confining. They were careful not to give me the idea that using a wheelchair was the end of the world (and it isn't) but even though their facial expressions masked their true feelings, the experience was still crushing. They were strong in front of me, but it really tore them apart inside.

It was hard getting used to using a wheelchair and it was equally hard being seen in one! I was at the age where appearance and doing the same things my peers were doing started to be very important. Fitting in was so desired. Learning to push myself was hard with the troubles that my right arm was giving me. Sitting was getting more difficult, so the chair was that much more restricting. And physical barriers popped up everywhere! Schools, sidewalks, stores, and other people's homes were difficult to get into and move around in. I was welcomed and assisted as a guest at someone's home, but no one else seemed to think it mattered that a person in a wheelchair could not access their building or establishment.

That summer we went on our family vacation. Before we left for the trip, my mom had contacted Dr. Tasker again because my condition continued to deteriorate. Plans were in the works for another trip to the Toronto General Hospital. Not knowing what the future would bring, we went on a special vacation to Disneyland. We saw San Diego, Anaheim (Disneyland) and Las Vegas. It was a wonderful, special time for the five of us despite an incident in the pool at our hotel in Disneyland. Before we left on this trip, I saw an advertisement for water wings— inflatable plastic flotation devices worn on the arms. I wanted them. I was probably too old or big to wear them, but they did the job. I began to love being in the water.

One day I was splashing around in the pool and two other girls that were my age came towards me. They inquired why I was using water wings. I simply told them I had a disease. They started screaming and swam for the stairs because they assumed what I had was contagious! Since no one else had ever responded in that manner, in a strange way it amused me more than anything.

While we waited for the date we'd fly back to Toronto, I needed extensive physical therapy daily. I found myself attending the Glenrose School Hospital for grades three, four and five. The only thing I liked about the physical therapy set-up was that an orderly came to my classroom at the same time every day, and I would miss a half hour to an hour of school. But I really disliked therapy because they wanted me to do things that were way beyond my limits. Therapy encompassed holding a normal position (such as kneeling on all fours), stretching, proper weight bearing, walking in parallel bars and more. Water therapy would come later. These tasks were more than I could do. It's not that I didn't *want* to do them, I *couldn't* do them.

My symptoms were so dominant that even if I could hold a position semi-normally, it would only be for a matter of seconds. When my muscles started to pull me out of position, my therapist would try to tap me back into place. That was a deal breaker, and my muscles would not cooperate even if they were able to help at all. I cannot force my dystonic muscles to move into any position that they do not want to be in! If it did work, it was merely a coincidence as far as I'm concerned and did not mean that my muscles were finally cooperating. Sometimes my muscles pull even harder in the other direction. Why did the therapist want me more frustrated than I already was? If I could do these things, wouldn't I be doing them on my own?

The Glenrose Hospital was an old rehabilitation hospital. The school was added on almost ten years before I was enrolled. Before the Glenrose built the school, disabled children who were deemed unable to attend regular neighbourhood schools could not attend school at all! So this school was a big deal for a lot of people.

It took a bit of getting used to. I was picked up and brought home on the Handi-bus, except on my first day at the Glenrose School. My mom drove and came in with me that day. We found Mrs. Paulson's classroom on the second floor. It was a small class—me and nine other students. The desks were small tables that could be adjusted for height so our wheelchairs could be driven right up to the table top. Only three of my classmates were not in wheelchairs.

A wide variety of disabilities were represented in that room: cerebral palsy (CP), muscular dystrophy (MD), spina bifida, mild learning problems, and paralysis caused by a gunshot wound. Bruce, the boy who sat in front of me had second – and third-degree burns. It was a bit of a shock when he turned around to look at me. He was small in stature, and his skin was bumpy and uneven. He had stubs for fingers, no external ear or nose cartilage and his mouth was more round than linear. He wore a baseball hat constantly because he had only one small tuft of hair at the base of his head. Donna, who had spina bifida, had little feeling in her legs so she had suffered severe burns from bath water that was too hot. Leonard, the boy with the gunshot wound, had been playing with a gun with a friend and the gun had gone off accidentally. He was paralyzed from the waist down and harboured a lot of anger. He went into tirades and would rip up his workbooks. Peter and Joanne were two new classmates with muscular dystrophy. Peter was mild-mannered and shy. Joanne was giggly and had four sisters, all of whom had muscular dystrophy. The two students with cerebral palsy were severely affected by the disease. Cerebral Palsy can affect the body, the mind, or both. These two individuals had severe physical challenges. Jason could not talk, but he had a built-in tray on his wheelchair. The tray held a board with numbers, letters and common phrases that he pointed to in order to communicate. Heidi could talk, but was extremely hard to understand. She too had a letter board but preferred to try talking. Many times a person would have to ask Heidi to repeat herself. Failing that, she would have to rephrase her sentence. As a last resort she would use her letter board. Heidi and Jason both used typewriters for any writing they had to do.

I was now exposed to all types of wheelchairs, braces, chair inserts, walkers, and other odd contraptions. They weren't totally new to me; when I was fitted for my shoe brace, I was at the prosthetics department. That is where braces, artificial limbs, and wheelchair inserts are made. Prosthetic departments have a distinct smell emanating from the glues and particles of plastics that have been shaved down in order to properly fit the prosthetic to the individual. They are smells that I have never smelled anywhere else. I actually like the smell.

I made several trips to the prosthetic department. On my right foot, I was still wearing a bulky metal brace permanently attached to my orthopeadic shoe. My mom and I would have to make a special trip downtown because orthopaedic shoes could only be found in one store in Edmonton. In those days, braces were so heavy they made walking more laborious instead of making it easier. After my right foot started acting up, it didn't take very long until other muscle groups started doing their own thing, going their own way, and totally throwing me off course.

Over time my doctors and therapists fitted me with a series of braces and other devices designed to keep me sitting or walking straight. Prosthetics are custom-made to meet individual needs, but my muscles never let me be comfortable in one position, unless it was an unnatural one, and the prosthetics weren't going to let me sit all twisted. My muscles won the battle. The doctors could try, but nothing they could fit me with could force my muscles into submission or normalcy. I've broken many braces, wheelchair footrests and inserts, a raised leg rest, and other devices. I've been known to bend steel. These muscles have power!

Chapter 10

In November of 1975, four months after "round one," our anticlimactic first visit to Toronto, we went back. The previous surgeries had yielded only temporary results. My movements were intensifying, so we thought we needed to try again. Dr. Tasker recommended doing the same thing as he had done before. He would locate the area he froze before and kill more tissue surrounding this area. Another preparatory surgery had to be done because my head had grown and the x-rays and measurements would now be different. This surgery went fine, but afterwards, as always, the anesthesia made me vomit and I had a fever. The perfect way to help bring down my temperature was to open the window and let the frigid November air flow into my room.

This time, while the doctors again operated on the left side of my brain to benefit the right side of my body, something went terribly wrong. During the thalamotomy surgery I was extremely spastic and could not lie still on the operating table. They gave me small amounts of drugs to calm me down, but I had still had to be aware of what was going on. Part of the success of the surgery depended on my telling them when the probe was in the correct area. This sedative made me sick to my stomach, so despite the fact my head was in a vise to keep my head completely immobile, they turned me on my side enough to vomit.

The surgical team found the area it was looking for, and Dr. Tasker started to freeze the area surrounding it. While doing so, a blood vessel was hit that caused a stroke on the right side of my body. I was awake while all this was going on, but I don't have any recollection of it happening. I had a stroke and was paralyzed on my right side. They put me back to sleep, and after I spent quite a while in the recovery room they took me to the neurological intensive care unit (ICU). It was late evening by this time. My mom had had a long, tedious, stressful day waiting for me to come out of surgery, so although she wanted to stay by my side, she was relieved that I would be monitored all night in the ICU. She needed sleep. She was exhausted and devastated by the outcome of the surgery, but after seeing me stable, peaceful and groggy she left the hospital in a slightly better state of mind. I don't remember much of that particular surgery so it was great that my mom had taken notes.

Within a few days the paralysis slowly receded. My leg recovered first. That was good, but of course it was very weak now. I could stand and weight bear a bit. After a few days they had me using a four-pronged cane so I could walk short distances. My arm was the last part to regain movement. I was not looking forward to the hard therapy that lay ahead, but I wanted to be as normal as possible so I had no choice.

My parents had been warned that during a thalamotomy there was a two to five percent chance of a stroke or other complications occurring. Two to five percent! They felt the risk factor was so low they hadn't given much thought to the idea of something going wrong. But this stroke turned out to be a godsend because the dystonic movements were drastically reduced. Now I needed to concentrate on regaining strength. In later years when I tried harder workouts to strengthen and make my right limbs more useful, I started to feel the dystonic tendencies, such as the turning in of my foot or hand. This led me to believe that the dystonia is dormant in that area of the brain, but if provoked it may come back. Limited use of my right side is acceptable to me.

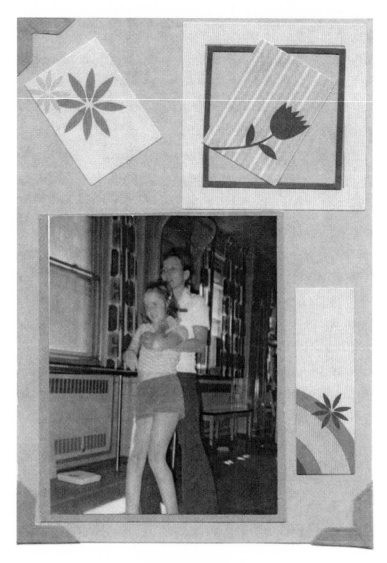

Ros and I in physiotherapy. 1976

I had physiotherapy daily. I loved my Toronto therapist, Ros, but I still hated physical therapy. Asking me to do something my muscles wouldn't let me do was beyond frustrating and bordered on being cruel, as far as I was concerned anyway. Usually whatever I was supposed to stretch didn't want to be stretched and so on and so forth. But since the stroke happened on the right side, at least I had a normal left side to support me and help regain enough strength to walk with a cane. That was hard, but I wasn't fighting stubborn muscles and I was getting some good results. Trying to exercise my right limbs after the stroke was a challenge that I didn't particularly want to face, but one I couldn't avoid. Before the stroke I always thought making the effort was useless and the struggle against the muscle activity was too great. After the stroke, I was encouraged to put more effort into it, but I was stubborn and didn't try very hard. My right arm was bent across my upper body, and my fist was still tightly clenched like it was before the stroke. When I pried it open it was always damp with sweat. Now, short stretches help and my arm and hand are more functional, but working the muscles back to a near normal state brings back those unwanted tendencies. The inward pulling and twisting, ever so subtle, of my right hand and foot scares the life out of me. It takes me back to the start of my ordeal. So I accept limited use of the limbs on my right side even though that has led me to overuse my left hand and arm.

Chapter 11

After the second round of surgeries, the stroke and the physical therapy, there was a time when I could walk. I was still in grade three at the Glenrose School Hospital. Occasionally I used my wheelchair since I wasn't quite ready to do the 100 yard dash, but I could use a cane or, if pushing someone else in a wheelchair, I could walk. Once, as I was going down the hallway at school in my wheelchair I passed a lady I didn't know. Later in the day I passed her again, but this time I was using my cane and walking. The lady asked me if I had a twin sister. Getting around in my wheelchair was easier because with my right side fairly silenced, my left arm and leg could propel my chair with ease.

Of course there were elevators in the Glenrose, some archaic and slow, but there was also a series of ramps connecting the basement and the main floor. One lunch hour, just to kill time, I pushed a classmate around in her wheelchair, and another girl, who could push her own wheelchair, came along. We decided to go to the basement via a ramp. If we went down one ramp and kept going, we could get to the older part of the Glenrose where the prosthetic department was located or we could make a 180 degree turn to go to the basement cafeteria, which was at the time, in the newer part of the Glenrose (The older part of the hospital has since been replaced). The cafeteria was our destination. At the end of this ramp was a cement wall. At that point we had to make a left 90 degree turn to reach the hallway. Me and the girl I was pushing managed the turn, but our friend who was pushing herself picked up speed, lost control, and went straight into the cement wall! She fell from her wheelchair to the floor and her two front teeth went completely through her lower lip. She had a couple more minor injuries. We were in trouble! But besides the injury to my friend, that type of lunch time activity was great exercise and did me a world of good.

Our family had grown accustomed to getting away in the summer. Retreating to a little cabin on a lake was more desirable than staying in a hot, noisy city for two months. Long drives to Shuswap lake were not going to be easy for me. Buying a trailer and having to pull up stakes at the end of our stay in campgrounds was not desirable either, so Mom and Dad decided to buy a lake cabin. In the mid-seventies they found a nice lake-front cottage on Lake Isle which is a one-hour drive west of Edmonton. The property needed a lot of tree and brush clearing. The cabin had neither power nor running water, so propane, kerosene lanterns, an outhouse and a fireplace got good use. Trisha and Kevin were often sent biking down the dusty road with empty plastic containers to fetch water from the public water pump. It would take a few years to make the cabin wheelchair accessible, so at first it was quite a struggle to get in and move around inside. The property was uneven, bumpy, and on a slight slant which made it quite a feat to move me around the yard too, but we had lots of fun nonetheless. Trisha and I loved to suntan although I got sunburned more often than not. Our transistor radio didn't get good reception when we tried to listen to our favorite songs of the day. Kevin had great fun teasing me with insects because he knew I didn't like them and feared some of them. After the first year or two there was a cycle of caterpillar infestation that lasted a few summers straight. Caterpillars were everywhere. They were falling out of tries, feasting on the leaves, traveling over roads in armies that made the roads slippery to vehicles. Nature could not have been any more horrific to me if it tried! My brother had a field day. I wasn't really an outdoor person at that point, so one summer I stayed inside every minute we were there. It is great that we now have power, water and phones out there, but I kind of miss the days when we had to rough it.

I had six months of near glory. I had learned to use a cane but sometimes I didn't need it at all. A weird quirk of dystonia is that some people can run but not walk forward normally. One overcast day out at the cabin I put on an old pair of my mother's rubber boots, went outside and started a brisk walk. It felt so good! I must have done twenty laps around our property without slowing down so as not to lose what I had going. Then one fateful day shortly after that, my mom's heart nearly dropped out of her chest. She noticed the movement and odd posturing was starting in my *left* foot!

Chapter 12

My left side was now involved in the battle. Our hope, with the limited knowledge that we had about the disorder, was that all I had to contend with was the challenges of the stroke. But we were wrong. My muscles were becoming more belligerent. My left foot was starting to clench, my hip and knee were extending and sometimes drawing up at an inward angle, and my lower torso was twisting to the right. My foot would not stay on the foot pedal of my wheelchair, and the rest of my leg would not stay in alignment with my trunk. My leg insisted (and still does) on pulling out and away from me. If I tried to walk in a walker I could not keep my leg from seeking the outer limits of the walking aid.

This turn of events showed us how aggressive this disorder could get, so Mom thought it best to be just as aggressive fighting back. She decided we should try the surgery again. Since they'd be working on the opposite side of the brain, it would be like starting with a clean slate. She knew I was afraid of having more of this surgery, but my muscle movement was dominating my life. The potential to regain control of my muscles, to have them relax and work normally, was something we had to try for. If I didn't try another surgery, we would always be wondering, *what if?* So, I reluctantly agreed.

On August 17, 1976, I was admitted to the Toronto General Hospital for the third time. This would be my longest stay: fifty-one days. Mom and Dad figured that if surgery was in the cards, my brother and sister should get a chance to see Toronto and visit me in the hospital. School was still out for the summer, so the timing was good. Kevin and Trisha waited to get a flight by student standby, the cheapest way to travel by plane at the time, and arrived a few days after Mom and I did.

It was great to have them there, if only for a short time. I was upset when Mom took them to the famous Canadian National Exhibition (CNE) without me. How dare they not take me? I got weekend day passes! Of course it was their time to bond and have fun without me, but it was still hard to accept. They didn't stay in Toronto for long. The first day of school was fast approaching, and they didn't want to miss the start of the school year. This upset my dad because he had sent them there for my mom's sake. School was important, but my parents gave them the chance to miss a few days for the benefit of us all.

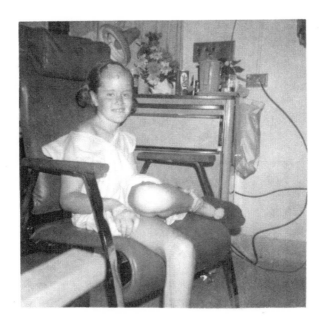

*After the 8th surgery my left leg was still
drawn up and inward. 1976*

By this time my condition was serious and my dad was
not handling it well. On the outside he appeared to be in
good spirits, but on the inside he was struggling. He did
not want to talk about the situation, which my mother
really needed to do. He would agree with the decisions
about surgeries, but that was about it. My mom wished he
had a close friend to talk to. She had many good friends
and she poured out her emotions and feelings to them.
But like most men, Dad did not do that. He was also
being very hard on my sister and brother. Their grades

in school were suffering. In different ways, dystonia affected everyone in my family.

Preparatory surgery was scheduled for August 30 and the thalamotomy for September 8. During this third visit to Toronto, which was the last visit to involve surgery, the second surgical complication took place. This thalamotomy was the first and last attempt to help my torso and left leg find peace. Prior to that surgery my left arm was the only limb unaffected by the disorder. We had expected it to progress into my left arm because that is what had happened on my right side. Because it hadn't happened, we counted our blessings. But things were about to change. Very quickly.

During this thalamotomy, on the *right* side of my brain, the probe most likely nicked the connections between my cerebellum (which controls the coordination of movements) and other motor areas of the brain. This resulted in tremor from my left shoulder to my fingers. Because of the complications caused by this surgical blunder, I was taken once more to the Intensive Care Unit.

Ever since I woke up after that operation (my ninth and final brain surgery) I have had tremors in my left arm, hand, and shoulder. My fine motor skills are limited because of the tremors, so everyday tasks like drinking from a glass and doing up buttons are challenging and sometimes impossible.

A Twisted Fate

Pre-dystonia I had been right-handed. As the disorder progressed into my right arm and hand, I had to make the change to the left. Considering everything else, that wasn't much of a problem. The big problem was now I had limited use of both arms. Each was affected in a different way, and I was worse off than I was before the surgery. My coordination was greatly diminished. I was very weak and could not do much for myself. When I was placed in a wheelchair, I had to be propped up with pillows. This was not at all what we had envisioned when we made the trip to Toronto, but we had to anticipate that something could go wrong again.

A day or so after that surgery, my mom phoned me early in the morning. I remember flailing about trying to reach the receiver, grip it, and bring it to my ear. When I managed to get near the phone, the receiver went flying. I was devastated because I was sure the person on the other end would not phone back. That was pretty silly since the majority of calls were from my mom, and I knew she would never give up that easily. She knew what was going on. She phoned back.

Another source of major frustration, among so many, was trying to use the earpiece for the television. Mom and Dad always made sure I had a TV and a private phone in my room. This was the '70s, when the hospital TVs were black and white, only got three channels and at least two of which needed constant adjustments. The only

(77)

way to hear was through an earpiece. The day before this surgery I had no trouble putting in the earpiece, but after that it was way beyond my control. The nurses and my therapists brainstormed and they tried threading the earpiece through the bottom of a Styrofoam cup and propping the cup up to my ear. It wasn't a great solution, but it was better than nothing.

I thought I'd had a lot of occupational therapy before that surgery, but I hadn't seen anything yet. It took time, but I now have more control of my left arm. The tremor is somewhat under control, but I still don't have the fine motor skills required to drink from a full glass, drink anything hot, or button up most clothing.

I use my left hand to do almost everything, mostly out of habit. That was fine for years, but now it is starting to put undue strain on my left hand and forearm. I still have to consciously remember to let my right arm take over whatever it possibly can to avoid the strain. Although using my right hand is a necessity, it still is quite the challenge. I am very much a creature of habit.

Chapter 13

The one constant in this unpredictable journey was my mom's support. Mom was always there when I got back from surgery. She usually had quite a long wait. Most times she was alone and went for long walks, weather permitting. She also picked up the hobby of crocheting to pass the time. She produced at least two sweaters and two bedspreads. After one surgery she bought me a stuffed animal—a dog made out of rabbit fur—to add to my collection. After another surgery she bought me a little Mickey Mouse clock. She was getting tired of me asking her the time every five minutes.

Although we could often see some sun through the cloudy sky, my mom was unsure whether our wider family network really understood how difficult this journey was becoming for us. The highs and lows of living and dealing with this strange entity were stressful to say the least. My mom had great friends to talk to, but they had no idea what it was all about either. But then again, how could they? For the first few years Mom had no one to talk to who was going through the same thing. Doctors could never say specifically where someone could seek out others with dystonia, so how were we to find them?

When I was at the Glenrose, we found out that there was one other student with dystonia, but they could not tell us who it was. There was one boy who had severe spasms and abnormal posture. He was in a wheelchair and could not talk. I always thought it was him. Many years later I saw him from a distance sitting in my neurologist's waiting room, so now I am fairly certain that this was the boy from long ago that shared troubles similar to mine.

My mom was personally hurt that I had to deal with these problems that, in all probability, would be with me as long as I lived. It was so hard to see other children my age being active and independent. I was a curious child who loved to be part of everything going on around me, and she knew I was taking that side of this disorder particularly hard. At some of my lowest moments, as consolation she would tell me again that, if they could, she and Dad would take this burden in my place. It is not easy sitting on the sidelines, watching others do certain things that I would love to do myself, but given time I have adjusted.

Mom debated whether it was easier to lose a child or have to see one battle a chronic, progressive, unpredictable disease that she was powerless to stop. She didn't think death was better, not by any means, just different. She didn't dwell on it though. She was positive that there would be a cure any day. If not today, then tomorrow!

Chapter 14

During our second trip to Toronto, my mom often went for strolls without me. On a few occasions she came back very excited because she had met someone of interest. One day she told me about meeting a fourteen-year-old boy named Chuck and his mom. He had dystonia too, but my mom didn't tell me that part right away. Chuck was severely affected. He was around ten years old when he started to show typical symptoms such as strange posturing of his foot that made touching the floor with his heel impossible. Within two years he was totally overtaken by dystonic movement. He could not sit or talk. His right arm repetitively flailed, rubbing against his head. His right eyebrow and a patch of hair on the right side of his temple had been rubbed away. We hadn't had much exposure to others with this disease, so Mom didn't let me know he had dystonia. She didn't want me to know, at my age, how much worse my dystonia could get. It can go anywhere at any time. Chuck still had a great sense of humour and a great smile. We grew quite close to him and some of his family members, especially his mom, one sister Joanne and one brother Bill.

Chuck's mom, Betty, had a tough life. She had nine children, and when the youngest was a toddler her husband was killed on the job. He met his demise while working for the Canadian Pacific Railway. He was loading piggyback units for trucks onto flatbed rail cars. One unit accidentally got loose and he was crushed beneath it. Chuck was already showing dystonic symptoms at the time of his father's untimely death. Chuck's mysterious, haunting symptoms, combined with the sadness and trauma of his dad's sudden death, made it that much harder for the family to cope.

Chuck, like many disabled people, loved to swim because of the freedom it afforded. The water's buoyancy provides a level of independence that cannot be achieved on land. Chuck frequently used a neighbour's swimming pool. His family looked into getting their own above – ground pool, but the company didn't have a design to meet their needs or budget. After finding out more about Chuck and his circumstances, the pool company offered to donate an in-ground pool if the family would dig out a form 14 feet wide by 26 feet long and 4 feet deep. It was a daunting task, but they recruited all their friends and within forty-eight fun-filled hours they had their hole and, soon after, the pool to go with it! They had a small back yard but were able to make it work. A sign stencilled on the changing room door read 'Chuck's Pool.' Chuck and his family became friends with us and had us over to their small, yet inviting home on more than one occasion.

Chuck had had numerous thalamotomies, but like me, he gained little relief from his symptoms. Because all those traumatizing procedures provided little to no help, his mom wondered if it was worth putting him through all that risky surgery. But in situations like ours, we try anything that will buy a little speck of hope and freedom.

Chuck's left hand was mobile enough to signal *yes* or *no*. He'd lift one finger for *yes* and two for *no*. I believe this was the only communication tool he had, but I bet his eyes and facial expressions told a lot to those who knew him best. Chuck, his sister Joanne, my mom and I had had some good times together killing time during the boring hours of sitting in a hospital all day and into the evening. One evening they got Chuck on a gurney and me in my wheelchair and we toured the halls. I tagged along holding on to the end of the gurney. We came to a point in the hallway where empty hospital beds sat on either side of the corridor. They steered Chuck's gurney between the obstacles, but I was not paying enough attention to guide my wheelchair between the two beds. My right hand could open enough to clutch onto things, but letting go quickly was not an option once my fist was clenched onto an object. I was still grabbing the gurney, and since I didn't have the foresight or ability to let go in time, I was yanked out of my chair face first onto the floor. I didn't really hurt myself, so we all broke out in laughter!

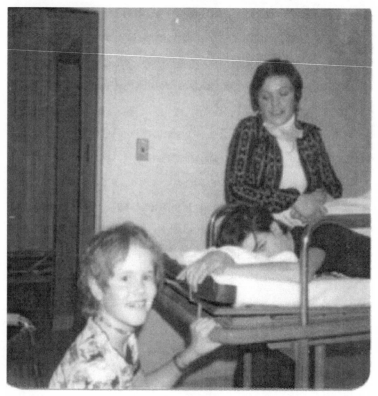

Me, Chuck and his sister Joanne venturing out in the halls. 1976

Another night, things were slow on the ward. We were in Chuck's room that had a window looking out to the hallway. His room was right across from the nursing station. There was a nurse sitting and doing paperwork. We knew this nurse had a great sense of humour. So Joanne, Chuck's lively older sister, rang his bell to summon a nurse. This nurse came quickly but found that Chuck didn't need assistance. She kind of laughed it off and went back to the station. Joanne and Chuck kept ringing the bell until the nurse finally had enough and came back with a roll of tape and excessively taped Chuck's hand to the bedrail!

There was a Marcus Welby connection to Chuck's diagnosis too! The day of my diagnosis the show featured dystonia on an episode called "Hell Lives Upstairs." Chuck might have waited a lot longer for his diagnosis, or never been diagnosed at all, if it weren't for that episode! One of his sisters happened to be walking by the TV room when the show was on, and she heard something that caught her attention. The symptoms described on this episode sounded similar to Chuck's, and that comparison led to his diagnosis. It was a big enough deal to wind up in a celebrity tabloid magazine. Just like my mom did, Chuck's mom wrote down the name of the New York doctor mentioned at the end of the show and contacted him the next day. She was told that they could get the diagnosis and surgery from Dr. Tasker, right there in their own city of Toronto. The family was honoured when they received a reply letter from actor Robert Young who played Dr. Marcus Welby, telling them he was very pleased that that episode had played a big part in getting Chuck diagnosed.

I don't recall exactly when I learned that Chuck's disorder was dystonia. I probably figured it out for myself since he had such uncontrolled movement and he too was having thalamotomy surgery also. But I certainly knew when we got the heartbreaking phone call in January 1978, when we were back in Edmonton, that Chuck had died of pneumonia. He had become so weak he couldn't fight it any longer. They had diagnosed the pneumonia too late to save his life. Chuck had not yet turned eighteen!

Later I learned that if dystonia affects the throat, it not only affects speech, it also makes it difficult to swallow. Food or liquids that should enter the esophagus, which leads to the stomach, can instead be aspirated into the lungs. This malfunction can easily bring on pneumonia.

Chuck meant so much to everyone. Of course his mother was most devastated by the loss. She had watched him suffer for years with indescribable helplessness. She wanted no more involvement with doctors or hospitals.

Chapter 15

During the long stays in hospitals I hated sitting in my room all day with little to do. It's different these days with computers, satellite TV, DVDs and video games to keep hospitalized children from complete boredom. We had TV, but in the '70s we only got two or three channels and most shows weren't of interest to kids. I didn't have anyone to phone locally, and Mom could only read to me for so long, so I continually asked her to take me strolling around our floor. We walked and walked for as long as Mom was up to it.

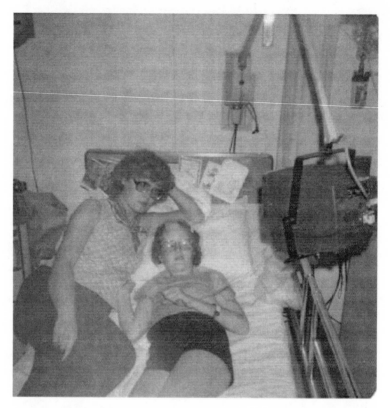

Mom and I. Killing endless amounts of time watching TV.

One day, when we were walking by one of the intensive care rooms, we saw someone sitting just outside the room in one of the hospital's signature green Naugahyde chairs. The change of scenery in the hallway offered more excitement and stimulation than the long days in the ICU room did. We stopped to say hello to the young man wearing a hospital gown. His name was Steve, and his mom was sitting with him. Steve was in his late teens or early twenties and had recently had surgery to try to remove a brain tumour. A fresh scar ran down the back of his shaven head and continued part way down his neck. It was disturbing to see. He told us a friend had come up to visit him, saw his scar, and had to make a quick exit to the bathroom! He was a good-looking young man and very polite. They were from North Bay, Ontario. We got very friendly with both him and his mother. The day I was discharged, we went to say goodbye to Steve, who was out of ICU and in his own room, to wish him the best of luck. He seemed to be in good spirits, and we smiled as we said our goodbyes. My mom knew he only had a short time left. Once again, we got a long-distance phone call. Steve had passed away five days after we had left for Edmonton. Until his final days he didn't tell anyone that the tumour had claimed his eyesight. He was blind the day we said goodbye, but he didn't mention it. His mom had given me two pictures of this handsome young man in better days. I am so glad she did.

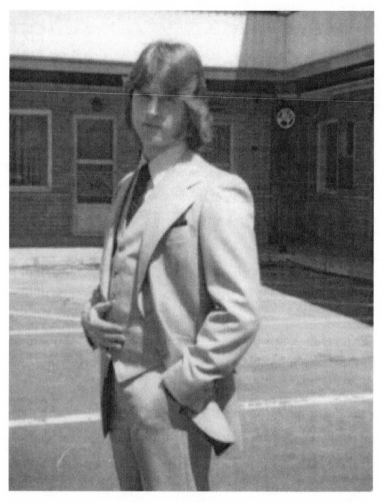

Steve, handsome and polite, before his brain tumour. Mid 70's.

Meeting people like Steve, Chuck, and their moms made walking the halls interesting and worthwhile. But most of the time, hall walking was monotonous. There was a little old lady who had to be tied to her chair whenever she sat in the hallway. Every time someone went by she would beg and plead with them to help her escape. There was a man who had an aneurism and declared himself a King. There were two young women who, because of aneurisms and brain injuries, were in vegetative comas. It was sad, but they were referred to as 'the twins.' One night a nurse took me with her on her medication rounds. We went into their quiet, still room to fill their feeding tubes. A feeling of great despair filled their room.

I dreaded hospital food, but at least I was conscious and didn't have to be tube fed. I was a small person at the time, and since I wasn't really active I ate very little. I admit to being a picky eater, but I'm less picky now. It seemed every time I was hospitalized I came out a little thinner than when I went in! My mom was a guest at someone's home, but she was with me for most meals. If she wanted to eat, she had go to the cafeteria and pay for meals. Through organizations that existed at the time, Mom could keep a list of expenses and get reimbursed for some of them, but she tried hard to keep her list down to a minimum. I was stubborn when it came to food, especially hospital food, so Mom knew I wouldn't eat what was left no matter how long it sat in front of me. I was the same way at home. Before we had a dishwasher, my sister and brother were often mad at me because we all had to do the dishes together. When I was made to stay in my chair until I ate my vegetables, they were often done while I was still at the table staring down at my untouched plate. My aversion to eating hospital food often worked out well: If I didn't eat much, Mom would finish off what was left. The nurses were so impressed that I had eaten all my food!

A nurse finally told me that I could pencil in hamburgers and milk shakes on the menu! The burgers weren't that great, but they were heads and tails above everything else. And you really can't go wrong with milkshakes. Where was this informant earlier?

I also discovered I had options when it came to taking medication. After the surgery that caused my stroke I was put on Dilantin, an anti-seizure medication. The nurses brought me this disgusting orange creamy liquid that tasted absolutely horrid. Most adults can suck it up and swallow without comment, but an eight year old? No way. Not me. Every time they gave it to me I complained profusely until finally a nurse said, "Oh, you don't like it? I can give you the capsule version." I ask again, "Where were these informants earlier?"

Chapter 16

On my third visit to Toronto, after I was admitted, we headed off to the ward. We were in the basement waiting for the elevator when a big, burly, middle-aged man approached me and said, "So you must be Brenda Currey. We've been waiting for you." I was perplexed as to how he knew who I was. I supposed a nurse from my previous stay had been talking about me and knew I was coming back. His niece, who was around my age, was on my ward along with another girl from Edmonton. I can only speculate that they both had cerebral palsy. His niece could speak well whereas the other girl could not talk at all. That was the only time I was aware that there were other children in the hospital and on the neurological floor while I was there.

This fellow's name was George, and he encouraged me to call him Uncle George. He was an actor—an extroverted man who was quite impulsive. The night before the surgery that left me with the tremor in my shoulder and arm, Mom had a rare opportunity to attend a pool party. There she could socialize with people that weren't doctors or nurses, have a glass or two of wine, and forget about our troubles and the hospital routine. She wanted to forget the fact, if only temporarily, that I was having surgery the next morning. Unfortunately, the evening was not as stress-free as she deserved. Mom decided to call me to say good night. I didn't answer my phone. After a few more times of calling my room and getting no response, she phoned my nursing station to ask where I was. After a quick look around the ward, the nurses could not find me or the other two girls. We were gone!

That night, Uncle George brought a few friends to help push the three of us girls in our wheelchairs. It was a beautiful evening, warm and humid. They took us for a walk. I remember walking through China Town. Roasted ducks and chickens hung from their feet in the merchants' store windows. Uncle George bought a few for us to try. The chicken was moist and tasty. We ate with our hands as we strolled. We also visited Toronto's City Hall. In front of this well-known building is a shallow pool with fountains set between two curved towers. To cool us off he put us, wheelchairs and all, into the pool! There was not much more than a foot of water, so our clothes didn't get wet, just our bare feet. We were in for just a few minutes. Then to top off the experience, we all got in a horse carriage and had a tour of downtown! It was a fun romp through a part of the city that I did not know well. Uncle George had neither asked nor told any staff that he had taken us, so the ward was frantic until we returned a few hours later. He was in big trouble! I didn't keep in contact with this man, but I remember a year or two later I saw this self-professed actor in an Old Spice commercial!

We went home two months later. After this third trip to Toronto, my condition was not stable. I now had to get my left arm under control, to the best of my abilities, and get my energy back. My right hand and arm were clenched and stiff, my left arm now had a bad tremor, and my left leg and pelvis were still straightening and twisting.

Feeding myself was difficult, and writing was nearly impossible. Working on improving those skills was a frustrating experience. Since I could no longer write I had to learn how to use a typewriter which was a long and challenging process. Watching two of my classmates, who also had to use typewriters, made the transition from pen to machine that much easier for me. I type quite quickly now, considering I can use only one finger on my left hand.

Dr. Tasker kept in touch with us and was always willing to help in any way he could.

After six months, and minimal improvement in my condition, we decided to go back east *again*. We didn't know what I might gain. We doubted surgery was in the cards, but we really needed to see Dr. Tasker and see what conclusions he could come to regarding further treatment. During my fourth trip to Toronto, which would turn out to be my last hospital stay in the Toronto General, Dr. Tasker told me I was the most baffling patient he had ever had! After giving my symptoms a lot of thought, he decided that more brain surgery was not the answer.

My overactive inner thigh muscles made my legs scissor together, which made it even harder for me to stand or keep my balance. My neurosurgeon thought it would be a good idea to see an orthopedic surgeon about this problem when we got back home. Dr.Tasker consulted an orthopedic surgeon who suggested a procedure that would release my hip adductors. They would slightly sever those muscles on the inside of my thighs to stop the scissoring problem. To test whether or not that would be a good option, they had an anesthesiologist give me a shot of anesthesia in each leg to temporarily shut down the muscle activity. They were excruciatingly painful shots. When these shots kicked in, I remember walking, with my mom's help, up and down the hallway. My legs were definitely weaker than normal, but the shots helped erase the muscle spasticity temporarily.

My left ankle was pulling upward with so much strength that it made the whole foot clench up and the toes turn under, so they decided they would do an elongation of my Achilles tendon at the same time. My parents decided to go along with this surgery. It was time for action of another sort. My brain surgery era had come to a close. I was just not getting the relief I needed. Now I was entering the era of orthopedic surgery!

Chapter 17

In September '77, within days of starting grade five at the Glenrose, I was admitted to the Royal Alex Children's Pavilion for the second time. I was to have the hip adductor and left Achilles tendon surgery performed by my new surgeon, Dr. Greenhill. He was an older English chap and very sincere. Being an orthopedic surgeon, he tried to understand my neurological condition as best as he could.

He explained that after this surgery he had to put full leg casts on both legs that would be kept apart by a wooden rod. I would be like that for up to three months, and then I'd wear splints like that at night for three months! That part concerned us, but obviously no one involved realized the toll it would take on my legs, especially my left, dystonic leg: my dystonic muscles would not tolerate being restricted in such an aggressive, long-term manner without repercussions!

Upon awakening from the operation in the recovery room, my legs, as expected, were fully casted from my upper thighs to my toes. I never did like the recovery room. It is not a great place to be when waking up after having general anaesthetic. As I woke up, the nurses always talked loud as if my hearing had been compromised. They asked me what my name was and where I was. When they finally left my gurney, they talked just as loud to the other patients in the room. All I wanted to do was go back to sleep.

The most significant difference between my situation and that of most people who need casts is that my legs were spread almost four feet apart. I don't think I was much more than four feet tall myself! This had to be done so that these surgically lengthened muscles would not automatically go back to the way they were. They needed a good long stretch in order for the surgery to do me any good at all. When they took me back to my unit on a stretcher, we ran into a problem. I couldn't fit through my hospital room door! They had to tip me on my stretcher at an angle to get me through.

Children say the strangest things, and I was certainly no exception. I was a very naive girl. I took most things literally, and I would follow directions to a *t*, never, ever wanting to be misunderstood or unapproved of. I was ten years old at the time. Mom had once, for whatever reason, commented that her mom caught her shaving her legs as a teenager and told her sternly that she shouldn't have done that because she was too young and the hair would grow back thicker. This story, for some odd reason, had stayed in my head. That is what I recalled her saying, but I could have misinterpreted being that I was so young. When I was being prepared for my surgery, the nurses slathered me down with a disinfectant of some kind that resembled drying blood. Then they went ahead and shaved my legs. The first thing I did after getting back to my room and successfully through the door was cry out in horror to Mom that they had shaved my legs. I saw my mom trying hard not to laugh while assuring me that that was okay.

I was in for a tumultuous three long months! My muscles waged a battle inside those casts. *Note to doctors! Never cast a dystonic limb! (Strong opinion only)* The muscles do not care that it is mind-blowingly crowded in the cast. They want to move, and this does not change just because you have tried to restrict them from moving! They will find another path to follow. I really don't know how I coped with that cast. I don't know if I could do it again.

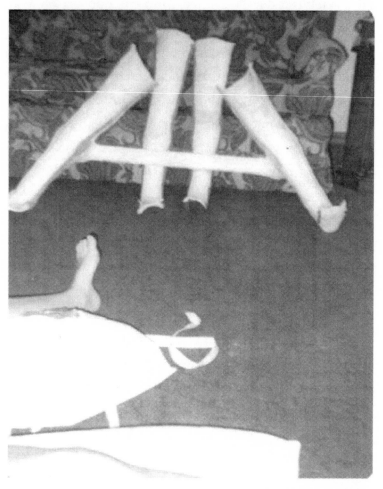

Check out my casts! How did I do it? 1977

For three months I spent nights on my back and daytimes on my stomach on a sponge – type wedge on a stretcher. Many times at night, to get relief from my muscles that desperately wanted to break free, I struggled to get up onto my left elbow, twisted my torso to that side, and lay on my bent arm. This usually helped me relax a little. My body just needed something different for a small distraction. Sometimes that would bring relief, but it was a lot of work! I would have fared a lot worse if I hadn't been taking Dalmane, a strong sedative, to sleep.

After a few weeks in the Royal Alex, I went across the street, via the underground tunnel, to the Glenrose where I would resume school and daily pool therapy. This time I was an inpatient on Station 201. I remembered always wanting to be a patient on Station 201. If you had to be a patient, this was the ward to be on! It was the inpatient rehab ward for students. In the days when nurses still wore white uniforms and nursing hats, the staff on 201 wore everyday clothes. Students who could not wheel themselves were personally escorted to and from the ward and the classroom. The older kids had a recreation room with a mini kitchen and a stereo system. During lunch hour and right after school, the stereo blared current hit albums such as "Fleetwood Mac." The music wafted down to my classroom in the adjacent hallway. There was a games room for the younger kids—the category in which I fit. The bedrooms and common areas were carpeted. It was trendier than the average hospital ward.

It's not that I didn't want to go home every day, but the prospect of riding the Handi-Bus for three hours a day did not appeal to me. I hated the name *Handi-Bus*;

it made me feel like a charity case! These were regular school buses, but only half as long as a standard school bus. There was space for four kids in wheelchairs at the back and seats for ambulatory kids. Hydraulic lifts were not widely used then, so the bus driver had to push a person in a heavy wheelchair up the ramp with just his own muscle power to rely on.

I got the raw end of the deal when it came to being bused to school. Although I did not live the farthest away, I was still picked up first in the morning and dropped off last in the evening. I lived in the west end of the city, and the Glenrose is north-centrally located. I was picked up at 7:30 a.m. and we proceeded farther west, then south, then east, and the final pick up was downtown. It would get quite chaotic in the Glenrose loading area with so many kids showing up around the same time needing help with jackets and other things. Going home, we retraced the morning route in the reverse order. It was an hour and a half each way, with loading and unloading time on top of that. It didn't make sense. I had a disorder that made sitting very uncomfortable and nearly impossible at times. Mom tried talking sense into them, but to no avail. Unfortunately, similar problems with disabled transportation still occur.

The ill-conceived idea of constricting my movement in full length casts caused more problems after the casts were removed. My right leg wasn't too bad while the cast was on because that was the side affected by my stroke. When the casts came off though, my right knee was so stiff I could not move it on my own. When a therapist tried to bend it, the pain was intense. My left leg was as active as ever while I was in the cast. With nowhere to go, the muscles would tug back and forth. As a result, the muscles responsible for bending my knee eventually raised my knee cap out of its natural position, which made bending an issue on the left side also. The problems caused by the cast incarceration made therapy a dirty word.

I was in those casts for six weeks before they cut the tops off of them to get me out of them for water therapy. When I was done, they put them back on and secured them with straps. Anyone who has ever had a cast taken off knows how freaky that procedure is. They use a drill with a round blade that looks like it will cut your leg off along with the cast, but somehow this instrument never cuts when it contacts the skin. It does not cut anything soft, and there are always a few layers of gauze between your skin and the cast.

It's an eerie feeling, a vibrating tingle. I felt so fragile when the casts were off after having been in them 24/7 for six weeks. I was out of them for an hour twice daily during water therapy. I could not bend my knees very far, so my new physical therapist, Debbie, moved them manually in the pool. It hurt immensely on both knees. I had combative, dystonic muscles to fight. Even if I hadn't had a procedure my muscles would still be combative and difficult to bend, but not nearly as much! I cried every time, but I think the crying was more out of fear of my kneecap breaking or other major damage being done. Oh, how I feared therapy!

One afternoon after pool time, an orderly was taking me back to class. The stretchers were not very wide, and I was always kept on my stomach on a foam wedge during the day. The stretchers did not have a lot of support for my legs that jutted out on either side. Upon entering the elevator, he lifted one of my legs to tilt me so I would fit through the elevator door. Off the other side of the stretcher I slid! He was very apologetic and whoever was passing by at the time helped him lift me back onto the stretcher. Then we proceeded back to my classroom.

My family was wonderful to me; they brought me home almost every weekend. It took a lot of strategy and effort, yet they still brought me home. I didn't fully realize at the time that bringing me home in my casts was such a difficult procedure. I was just happy to be going home. They borrowed a friend's station wagon but, even in this car, one leg had to go up onto the wheel well so I was tilted the whole ride home! Being packed sideways to get me through the back landing and up the three stairs was problematic to say the least. When I was inside the house, they picked a spot in the living room where I stayed practically the whole weekend. On occasion they hauled me downstairs where our only TV was located. That required skillful maneuvering. It was great to sleep in my own bed even though it was still awkward.

Chapter 18

I had a whole host of roommates over the years, but I was truly blessed when I was on Station 201 for the first time. I made a great friend named Theresa. We were in a four-bed hospital room and her bed was kitty-corner to mine. We got along well and became fast friends. She was two years older than me, but that didn't matter as is often the case with kids. Theresa was from the small city of Red Deer, Alberta which is about an hour and a half drive south of Edmonton. Her parents often made the journey from Red Deer to bring her home. On some weekends that she didn't go home, she came home with me. She was such a delight to be around, and my whole family enjoyed having her. We had a prepubescent crush on teen heartthrob Shaun Cassidy at the time and had matching t-shirts with his picture on the front.

Theresa suffered from serious and painful juvenile rheumatoid arthritis. She was diagnosed when she was only sixteen months old and required intensive physio-therapy and water therapy that was not available in her home city. She was a real ray of sunshine—smart, cute, positive, giggly—and very wise for her age. I can only imagine how painful her arthritis was, but I never heard a complaint leave her lips. In later years, I believe she had a hip replacement, a jaw/chin replacement (because her chin had not fully grown with the rest of her face) and several other surgeries.

Since she lived in Red Deer, we didn't see each other very often after we left the Glenrose, but we would write occasionally. She attended the University of Alberta (U of A) and became a pharmacist. She wasn't married yet, and she knew she may always have to support herself. While studying at the U of A she spent some weekends with us again. She considered my mom and dad her parents away from home.

Her happiest memories had to be her wedding and then the birth of her daughter. She researched arthritis and motherhood and found that other women with her condition had healthy children. She and her husband decided that was what they dearly wanted, and she had their daughter, Lauren, in 1997. Fortunately I was able to visit her in person in May of 1998. But unfortunately, shortly after that, she broke her arm after tripping over a cord at the pharmacy she worked at. Her arm was not healing like it should. While she was at the hospital exploring the possibility of getting the bone fused, a blood clot developed in her system. She was treated quickly, and they were able to save her. But three days later, in the hospital, after having a fun evening playing and bonding with Lauren, another clot developed while she slept. She died instantly. I'm so glad she came into my life. I will not forget the sound of her voice, her cute little laugh, and her valued friendship.

Chapter 19

During grade five at the Glenrose, after my surgery and cast ordeal, Dr. Greenhill suggested I go back to a regular public school for grade six. My eyes lit up with interest. It sounded great, but it wasn't going to be easy. This was before integration was anywhere near mainstream yet. We couldn't have imagined how hard the Edmonton Public School Board was going to make it for us.

The first battle was approaching schools. The school that I attended for grades one and two, Meadowlark Elementary, first told my mother that I was welcome to come back for grade six. So Mom set up a meeting with the principal, who was new and had not met me. My mom also had my physical and occupational therapists and my current teacher attend to work out any kinks that might arise. But the school had recanted its decision. Apparently this principal had talked with the people at the Glenrose, and suddenly there were all sorts of problems. I do not think that the Glenrose had deliberately tried to discourage this school from taking me in but the principal had given my limitations more thought and decided against letting me attend. There was the possibility that I might fall while using my walker or distract the other students with the noise from my typewriter. My mother was stunned by that decision and left the meeting in tears. She approached all the other local public schools in our area, but they all reacted pretty much the same, much to our chagrin. The rejection from Meadowlark—where my brother and sister had gone for all six years of their elementary education, and I had gone for my first two—took its toll. The last school that she approached half-heartedly said I could attend, but it didn't feel right and my mother didn't want to send me somewhere she knew I was not wanted. To them I was considered a total liability.

I think the Glenrose didn't want me to go because they didn't think I could keep up with my peers. I believe that one hang-up they had was I had fallen behind because of the time I was away during my hospitalization and the classes I missed twice daily when I was having water therapy. Oh, how I worked on catching up! I had workbooks to finish and I worked very hard at my homework every night, awkwardly clicking away at my archaic typewriter. I had something to prove! What was so wrong about this situation was that these schools never asked about my abilities or accomplishments. When I was attending the Glenrose I took an IQ test, and I was above average!

Finally my physiotherapist, Debbie, suggested we try approaching Catholic schools. We weren't Catholic, but I didn't have to be in order to attend. The principal at the first school we approached, Our Lady of Victories, welcomed me with open arms. The principal told us I would be good for the other children and vice versa. The situation was perfect because it was a one-floor school and close to our home. To them I was considered an asset!

I never injured myself or anyone else, and over the course of seven years not one complaint was made about distractions due to my typewriter or anything else. To add to the goodwill from the Catholic School Board, they provided cab rides to and from school every day for the rest of my school days!

My mom wrote the following letter to the principal of Meadowlark School, soon after the disastrous meeting, but she never did send it:

May 17, 1978.

Dear Principal,

I went home today and told a beautiful little girl that her first school, Meadowlark, turned her down. I will never forget the look on her face, nor will I forget my next words to her. "Don't worry honey, we will try and find another school willing to accept your physical handicap."

I am not bitter with you and your staff, but I am most certainly disappointed. Brenda has come a long way in the past four years. She is a brave little girl and has more courage than most of us. The most disappointing point to me is that you were not willing to give Brenda a chance, a chance that she wants to take. She is keenly aware of the problems that lay ahead. We have crossed many hurdles in the last four years, and it looks like this is going to be our most difficult one. Brenda has had six major brain operations, and a major operation cutting nerves and muscles in her legs. She has overcome a stroke and has had years of physiotherapy. She has become stronger after each time.

You at Meadowlark will be the losers. Brenda has much to offer your staff and your students. Strength, Courage, Conversation, Charm, a sense of humor and most of all Love.

Brenda and all the many children like her are people not just somebody who cannot walk or write quickly and neatly. They should be with children their own age, not with people who are all physically and mentally handicapped. They must be motivated with children their own age. Brenda is bright and alert, and wanted to be in her own community.

I thank you for your time today, and I am sorry that I could not control my feelings. You must climb the mountain to get to the other side. I will just keep climbing, and with God's help I will make it.

Yours Truly,

Mrs. Sheron Currey.

At that time in my life I had mixed feelings about the Glenrose school hospital. They had made it more difficult to get out into what I called "the real world," but now I remember my time at the Glenrose as the biggest learning tool I could have ever had. I was exposed to the human condition and to people who had far greater problems, some of which were life-taking, disorders. But putting that aside, most were just happy children and teens. The school had a student council, field days, Easter Teas, Christmas concerts, Halloween and Valentine's Day parties, an awards night, and other events just like any other school. But we also had a physical and occupational therapy department, a pool, and a hospital ward. Doctor's clinics were situated nearby. The Glenrose has turned out many intelligent and successful people living within seemingly incapacitated bodies.

For the three years that I attended the Glenrose, even during the tense times near the end, Mom did volunteer work there. She had a few friends donate their time also. They were in the classrooms as teacher's aides or in the cafeteria assisting students who needed help eating lunch and cleaning up. She began to fully realize how limited most of these children were. Most were in heavy wheelchairs that did not allow them many choices about where they could go or how to get there. These children did not have the chance to run around during recess to work off any excess energy like able bodies could. Time spent outdoors was probably limited to their back yards—if they had one. There were not many chances to get away from the routine of being disabled. So near the end of each school year Mom convinced the Glenrose staff to donate the use of a Handi-bus to take my class to our backyard for a picnic. Mom spread blankets on the grass and anyone that wanted to get out of their wheelchair was helped to do just that. We always had good weather and lots of picnic foods!

At the end of grade five, which was my last year at the Glenrose, my mom had the idea and big job of convincing the school hospital to provide a Handi-bus to take us all out to our lake cabin for a day, an hour's drive out of the city. After a bit of skepticism, she got the go-ahead. Most of these children never had a chance to get out of the city, sit by a lake, or go for a boat ride. Fortunately we had good weather again, because our cabin was small and not wheelchair accessible at the time. I'm sure my mom had a backup plan for that day.

Everyone was helped into our ski boat and taken for a ride or two if they wanted. It was a new experience for some; the wind going through their hair and the misty water landing on their skin. We roasted wieners and had lots of chips and pop. It was quite the experience!

One of my classmates, Peter, was a small, shy and very weak boy who was fighting muscular dystrophy. In a thank you note to my mom following that day he wrote:

> 'Dear Mrs. Currey, It was a good day at the lake. It was fun going on the boat ride. I liked the cabin and the dog but sincerely didn't like the flies one bit', Sincerely peter.'

My fifth grade teacher, Mrs. R, also wrote a note:

> 'Dear Sheron, Thank you so much for a most pleasant day. Peter had a most serene look with a brilliant sparkle in his eye on the way home. It was much appreciated by all. Sincerely, Mrs. R.'

That was music to my mother's ears. That was exactly why my mom had made the effort to bring some 'normalcy' and a break from routine to my classmates.

Chapter 20

I was very nervous the first day of grade six at my new school because I didn't know if I would be accepted by my classmates. I feared rejection and teasing from the other kids, but everything went great. They had already set up a table for me to work at, with ample space for my typewriter, as well as a regular desk if I preferred to sit in it. I loved it there and thrived that year. We had a class clown that kept the class in stitches. My mom, at our minister's suggestion, contacted the *Edmonton Journal* newspaper and told them the story of the difficulty I had being accepted by the public school system and how it had worked out for the best at a Catholic school. When the article came out, the headline read "School a Joy for Plucky Brenda." I embarrassed extremely easily and was mortified because I didn't know what *plucky* meant. It didn't sound very dignified, so I was relieved to find out what it meant: courageous, determined, cheerful, spunky, and spirited. The article was good.

The hardest part of the whole year was walking from the vehicle to my classroom. I alternated between using my walker and my wheelchair. I was encouraged—or more accurately, forced—to use my walker for the exercise. Walkers had always been difficult for me to use because my left hip and torso pulled the left leg outwards. I could not stay within the parameters of the walker; therefore, most of the weight and strain was put on my right leg, which was still weak from my stroke nearly four years earlier. Using a walker places demands on one's arms, too. My right arm was extremely weak, so that support was also lacking. My right ankle muscles were so weak I had to wear a plastic brace on my right foot. My weak thigh muscles could not completely straighten my knee, so the inside of my right foot dug into the brace and created a big callous in that area. One can only exercise and strengthen limbs so far when the other limbs are not capable of doing their supporting role. My right leg, affected by the stroke, was now expected to carry my weight and counteract the insanity of my left leg? Using a walker was beyond tough!

I was very blessed to be taken to school in a taxi at no cost to my parents, but whether I took my wheelchair or my walker some cab drivers were a bit on the lazy side. Many would throw my chair or walker into the trunk and take off without closing the trunk. Some would not fold my walker down, which was a very simple thing to do; therefore, the trunk was left wide open. When we approached the school parking lot I turned twenty shades of red. It was extremely embarrassing at the time. It felt like instead of people thinking, *Here comes Brenda,* they thought, *Here comes Brenda and her impairment for all to see.*

My grades ranged from six to nine on a scale of one to nine. The last day of classes in grade six was sorrowful to me. I couldn't attend the junior high school that everyone else was going to due to accessibility issues. I had grown close to my classmates. One boy noticed tears in my eyes as I wheeled to the door to be picked up by my mom. He asked me what was wrong, and I blurted out that I may never see any of them again. I was loaded into my mom's car and, as we left the parking lot, my whole class poured out of the school waving and shouting goodbye! I attended Catholic schools for the duration of my school years—cab rides included!

Chapter 21

My mom nearly always had a part-time job despite her busy schedule with me, our family, and all her other duties. She was always home until my bus or cab drove away from our house. One rare morning she had to leave before my ride showed up. Our home had three cement steps at the front door. I would either awkwardly walk the three steps—with a lot of help—or I would be bumped up or down in my wheelchair. On this day, with my mom already gone, a female cab driver showed up. She decided to bump me down the three steps. On the last step she lost control and I was falling backwards. She could see that my head was going to hit the cement stair, so she put her arm under my head to soften the blow. My head was fine, but her arm was broken! We now realized we needed to have a ramp at the front door.

The cab driver wasn't the only person who ended up with a broken limb that year. Near the end of the school year, my left femur (thigh bone) was twisting inward and growing that way. If I was ever going to walk again, this would cause a significant problem. Dr. Greenhill decided that I needed to have it surgically broken and reset. We had just gotten back from our family trip to Hawaii, our last family holiday together because my brother was graduating from high school that year. I was at my new junior high school, St. Mark, working on a group assignment during lunch hour when my mom and dad walked in the room. I knew that meant a bed had become available at the Royal Alex. I burst into tears. I was enjoying school so much.

During this surgery, doctors broke and reset my femur and then attached a metal plate with screws to keep it in place. I remember declining the opportunity to view the x-rays! One thing that might have been nice, even though it wouldn't have changed anything, was being informed *beforehand* that they would be removing approximately one inch of the bone. My left leg already appeared to be shorter than the other because my left pelvic region had risen over time from the constant upward pulling of the muscles involved. I was already out of alignment, and now it was worse. Once again I was put in a body cast, although this time it encapsulated my left leg—the active one—and my torso.

After a number of weeks in the Royal Alex, I was taken again—cast and all—to Station 201 in the Glenrose. I was put in a temporary class because I would only be there for a couple of months. Again, being in the cast was very

difficult. It actually cracked at the hip and had to be fixed.
Again my left knee took the brunt of the six-week ordeal.

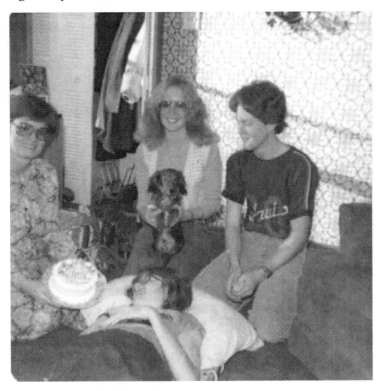

Plopped in the living room for my 13th
Birthday party March 1980

Water therapy was back in the picture. This time,
when Debbie tried to bend my left knee, I felt a lot of
pressure on my femur where the plate was located. I was
sure something was going to snap or rip apart if she bent
it hard enough. From the constant friction in the cast, my
knee cap had risen again. To bring it back down I would,

at a later date, need more surgery to slightly sever and lengthen the muscles involved.

Chapter 22

I had a wonderful friend named Ed who was once my horseback riding teacher when I was a member of the Little Bits Riding Club: a group founded for disabled children. At the time I loved horses. As soon as I heard about the club, I was eager to join. Disabled kids and teens had an hour of class time and an hour of riding the horse. It was great therapy, but every rider had to have a side walker: someone walking beside them holding onto the waist harness. With my unnatural posture I always appeared to be falling off, but that wasn't the case. The side walker would constantly pull on the harness to get me centered. This tug of war wasn't going to have a winner. No matter how good their intentions were, it was a battle.

My friend Ed was such a giving and larger-than-life person. He taught school in Africa for a few years and then found himself in Nicaragua helping the poor, defenseless, disabled street children. He came to visit me one night at the Glenrose. I don't know if he cleared it with the nurses, but he had a baby goat with him! We were in a common area of the ward, so anyone could come up and see or pet him. The goat was lying partially on my cast and decided it was time to take a pee—on me and my cast!

Ed is gone now having lost a hard-fought battle with cancer. He certainly will always be remembered by me and all the others who knew him. The world will miss him because his love and efforts reached around the world!

Chapter 23

My legs are very skinny. After the femur surgery, some extra padding on my thighs would have been very useful. After recuperating from surgery and the cast ordeal, lying on my left side was uncomfortable. For a few years after that surgery, whenever I lay on that side my leg fell asleep or went numb around my scar. You could actually see a small bump protruding from the top of the five-inch scar. It took me quite a while to convince my doctor to go back and take the plate out. I had to almost beg, but I literally had "a screw loose." Finally they did the surgery and it was no longer uncomfortable to lie on my favorite side.

My left knee cap was still a problem. I could not bend my leg very well, and the kneecap had risen again while in cast captivity. Again it took a while to convince them to do something, but finally they performed a quadriceps release. The muscles involved with raising my knee cap were slightly severed so it could ease back down to where it should have been. I could finally bend both knees to full capacity with no pain or discomfort!

While I was in junior high I had yet another surgical procedure; this one involved my toes. The constant curling under of my toes was one of the things that threw me off balance. Imagine that the muscles in one of your hands involuntarily took over, that it made a fist for so long and so strong that eventually one of your knuckles dislocated itself. That is what happened with my left foot, so once again some muscles were partially severed to release my toes' flexor tendons. It did not make much of a difference, but at least it wasn't major surgery so I was not hospitalized for long. I recuperated in days instead of months.

My left foot has been a great source of stress. Whenever I put my shoes on, my dystonic muscles, consciously aware that they are going to be restricted, fight back. My foot clamps up like a hand makes a fist. Most mornings my mom and I hated the shoe routine. Everyone else was out of the house by that time. Shoehorns did not work, so the ensuing struggle was physically and emotionally draining for both of us. Shoes at that time weren't made for comfort, and they didn't open wide enough to make it easy for a cramped-up foot to get in. The surgery had helped very little.

Although the shoe routine was frustrating and draining, it certainly wasn't the only reason we got emotional.

A Twisted Fate

Every morning when I got on the bus or in the cab, Mom always stood smiling and waving from the door until the vehicle drove away. I was unaware that many times my mom would go back to bed and cry as soon as she was alone in the house.

There were many reasons why my mom shed tears. Being my caregiver on top of the usual motherly duties was draining. Helping me dress and eat in the morning took time away from her own routine. She did some investigating and found an organization that paid half the costs involved with hiring someone to help me with my morning routine. Mom certainly deserved this break.

Chapter 24

My competitive nature has waned through the years. But when I was younger, I was very competitive whether I was playing games, selling raffle tickets for school projects, entering contests, or vying for the best marks at school. I remember a remark written on my year-end grade one report card that said I passed with flying colours. I wondered why it didn't say that on my grade two year-end report card, so my mom pointed out that I was in Toronto for part of that year. At anything of an academic nature, if I wasn't at the top I was always close to it. In grade seven, just before I was hospitalized in January for the femur surgery, I learned I had made the honour role. I was very pleased. On the same day that I came back to school, after more than six weeks in the hospital, my name was being removed from the display at the front of the school that listed who was on the honour roll. New report cards had just been issued, and unfortunately I hadn't made it for that quarter. Privately I was upset because they hadn't even given me a whole day of proudly seeing my name on the coveted honour roll board.

Whatever award was available I tried very hard to get. As my last year of junior high came to an end, awards night arrived. In past years I had not won any awards and had always been disappointed. Major disappointments always crushed my entire being, so although there was a new award being given out that year, I tried not to get my hopes too high that I would win it. It was the last award presentation of the evening, so when our vice-principal (VP) got up to the podium I blocked out much of what he was saying by looking around the gymnasium and wondering who the winner would be. There were a couple girls I was always in academic competition with, so I was sure it would be one of them. I heard snippets of his speech—"Every day she greets people with a big smile no matter what"— but I still didn't think he was talking about me. Hearing my name called out broke me out of my reverie. I had just won the Spirit of St. Mark Award for Great Courage! I hadn't caught on to the reason my brother and paternal grandparents were in attendance— until then. When I called back a year later to see when I should return my trophy, the VP said to keep it because it had never been given out before and would never be given out again.

The Dystonia Medical Research Foundation (DMRF) gives out Courage Awards every year. My mom submitted

A Twisted Fate

my name in the fall of 2001, and I was one of ten people who won this award for living life with great courage despite having dystonia.

Chapter 25

This disorder makes doing many things extremely awkward and clumsy. Well I was born into the right family for that! My brother was, and still is, a chronic teaser of his two sisters. Shortly after I was in my first wheelchair, Kevin found it great fun to terrorize me in it. Our driveway was on a slope, so he would push me to the top, facing the garage, and let go. My chair would slowly descend, swing around and pick up speed going down the slope. Then he would push me down the alley, picking up speed while I screamed at the top of my lungs. One day one of the small front wheels hit a big rock at the end of our alley. I went flying onto the pavement and acquired some scrapes on my legs. My mother was horrified. After expressing her concerns about the possible consequences for me had I broken any bones, she sent Kevin to his room. Even after that, whenever he pushes my wheelchair up and down curbs I sometimes believe he's forgotten I'm even there, for they are bumpy rides. And one time while we were out at the lake, we were walking along the side of a dusty road, and of course we were going too fast. He hit a rock with the front tire again and that catapulted me into a prickly Alberta wild rose bush!

I appreciate anyone's effort to give me a helping hand, especially my dad's. The people that I depended on and worked closest with were my immediate family. My dad's efforts to get me into a car resulted in my appearing less than ladylike! When my left hip and knee were belligerent and would not bend, he literally took me under my arms and threw me in the car feet first. His size, 6 feet 3 inches, and strength worked in his favour. As I got bigger my dad could not carry me in his arms anymore, so he started using the piggyback technique when the need arose. Normally this involves wrapping one's arms around the neck of the other person (the carrier) and wrapping the legs around the carrier's back. The carrier holds onto the legs securely so the person being carried doesn't fall. We couldn't do it the normal way because my hip would not bend. Since I couldn't wrap my legs around his body, it was up to me to hold on to his neck tightly enough short of choking him but not so loose that I might let go and fall off. I had to piggyback at my own risk. These methods seemed undignified, but realistically they were the best ways to do things at the time.

Vehicles have always been a thorn in my side. There is hardly ever enough room for comfort in either the front seat or the back. I am not claustrophobic, but my left foot, leg and hip are! I've had some extremely nightmarish car rides during which my hip screamed to straighten out and twist, and the rest of my muscles tried to follow suit in a compact area. Add the seatbelt and the nightmare is complete. My comfort level depends on the type of car, the height of the seat, the amount of leg room, and other variables. There is not much to do or say in that cramped environment, so I usually suck it up. Not every ride is a problem, but they happen often enough!

Most teenagers dream about getting their driver's license as soon as they turn the legal age of sixteen. It is the next step toward growing up and gaining independence. I was no different. I realized I had movement issues, but the Glenrose hospital offered disabled driving training. My mom did not discourage me from aiming for the goal of driving; she often let me drive down the back alley. I wasn't good, and I needed more practice. I had managed to get my learner's permit because that is based on a classroom exam. I got an appointment to be assessed at the Glenrose, and shortly after that my lessons began.

The instructor drove to an empty parking lot and we switched seats. I sat behind the hand controls. It was a rainy day, and the parking lot was full of pigeons. Before I had even turned one corner, my instructor told me then and there that I would never drive. She revoked my learner's permit on the spot. She may as well have pulled my heart out of my chest. I told her she had ruined my life, and I left in tears.

It took me a long time to get over that personal trauma. Not long after that experience I was at a family function and my brother arrived in his new sports car. A cousin of ours, who is a few years younger than I am, asked Kevin if she could take his car for a spin. He said yes and they drove away. Again, my heart was hurt and jealousy rose high within me. For the next few years, whenever younger friends or family members got their license, I felt jealous. Slowly I got over it, and now I'm actually happy not driving—with some exceptions. I knew in the back of my mind I never would drive, but when it meant so much to me I did not want to acknowledge the truth. Disabled transportation is still a huge waiting game, but I am grateful to have it.

Chapter 26

I credit my friend Jana for making my pre – and early teen years 'normal' for me. We met at church. The summer before grade six, my mom enrolled me in our church's day camp. When Jana volunteered to push me home the first day, we discovered she lived right across the street. My mom was so pleased. None of my close friends lived nearby so she kicked my butt to jump-start a friendship with this neighbour. Soon after that we did everything together. She was undaunted by my wheelchair and didn't hesitate when barriers arose. She carried me piggyback up or down any set of stairs. We did the teen grooming things like popping zits and trying to achieve the feathered hairdo that was the rage in the late '70s and early '80s. My hair would never do it. We went to movies, sporting events, the mall, sleepovers and church activities. I was often stared at by kids in the mall so sometimes we couldn't help saying that adolescent phrase 'Take a picture. It lasts longer!'

I have done my share of stupid and dangerous things in my life, but I think I have the number one, hands down winner here. When we were about thirteen years old, Jana and I were at my parent's cabin one summer weekend. Neighbours across the gravel road asked us over to their cabin one evening to sit around the bonfire and visit. The teenage son and a friend of his were our hosts. I was by the fire in my rickety old wheelchair, a spare chair that I used at the lake. I was positioned parallel to the fire. That was the first mistake. Then, because my body twisted to the right it was much easier to reach things on the right side of my wheelchair with my left hand. There was no table to put my glass upon, so my drink was on the grass to my right, between me and the bonfire. (Can you see where I'm going here?) While Jana and the boys were elsewhere replenishing the snacks, I bent over and reached for my drink. Next thing I knew I was in the fire! It all happened quickly. Fortunately the others were just exiting the cabin and could see what had happened. They quickly pulled the chair off me, rolled me in the grass, and hosed me down. I was lucky they had a water hookup with a hose—not many cabins did at that point in time.

I was in shock. What really saved me from any serious burns that frightful night was my hairdo and my clothing. My long red hair was done up in French braids, otherwise my whole scalp may have gone up in flames. And I was wearing a hockey jacket that had an asbestos lining that prevented my upper body from being burnt. I came away from this event with a cut on my neck that looked much worse than it really was (it didn't leave a scar), a tiny burn near my mid-section, and a wound slightly larger than a 25-cent coin on the inside of my left wrist. It got infected, but after a quick visit to the emergency room where it was treated with ointment, it was well on its way to healing.

I was very lucky after doing such a dumb thing. The strangest thing about that evening was my mom's premonition. She went to bed shortly after Jana and I went to the neighbour's, and every time she closed her eyes, she saw me falling into a fire. She just brushed it off until a bit later when there was a knock on the door and she got the news that I had fallen into the fire! God was certainly looking out for me on that summer night!

Jana's friendship surely was a gift. Unfortunately, with the onset of high school life, we drifted apart. We reconnected years later and are good friends again.

Chapter 27

These days, wheelchairs and other mobility aids are designed to be much lighter and user-friendly, but for many years of my struggle the chairs were heavy and hard to use. Now chairs are fitted more to meet an individual's needs, which is better for comfort and function. Accessibility to public places and their washrooms have come a long way also, although people designing buildings for public use might want to consult a disabled person or two before drawing up the plans. Better ramps and disabled bathroom stalls are at the top of the list!

Before the improved designs came along, repeatedly lifting a wheelchair that weighed over fifty pounds into the trunk of a car was physically demanding. It caused chronic hand, shoulder, and back pain for my mom and others. In addition to lifting the wheelchair, my helpers had to pull me from a sitting to a standing position—a challenge all its own—because my hip and knee resisted bending with the natural flow that comes so easily to most people. My mother has never said or done anything to insinuate that her pain was caused by me or my equipment, but I believe it was.

My wheelchair's foot rests were metal, but my muscle strength put so much pressure on them that I would bend or break them fairly often. Another problem I have with wheelchairs is my foot always hangs over the left side because my left leg will not bend unless I'm sitting at an awkward angle. The potential for injuring my foot and ankle is always present. No matter what type of foot rest I use, my left leg finds a way to avoid staying in the designated area of the foot rest. After all these years I have not hurt my foot or ankle. I instinctively know how to avoid trouble.

There are many things a person has to worry about if they have mobility problems. Most of the time I didn't have the coordination to push myself in a manual wheelchair, so I was dependent on someone to push me around. In junior high school I always had to ask a classmate for a push from class to class for I had no #1 friend who would volunteer automatically. I was very grateful the year I got my first electric wheelchair! I was in grade eight, and the freedom it gave me was long overdue.

Getting this electric wheelchair was wonderful, but I could only use it when I was at school. Because of its weight and size, there was no way to transport it back and forth from school to home. That left me dependent again when I wasn't at school. Transportation for people with a disability was available, but I was too young to use their services. When I had my power chair at home for the summer, I still had limitations. I could use it in my neighborhood and venture to the nearest mall, but that was about it. Curbs and other obstructions had not been recognized as significant barriers to people using wheelchairs at the time.

One Good Samaritan's efforts went awry one summer day as I set out to go to the mall on my own. I was having trouble with a curb cut that was still too high for my electric wheelchair to scale. While I attempted a different approach, a passenger in a car at a red light saw that I needed a hand. He jumped out of his car, asked if I needed help, and before I could answer he gave me a super shove up onto the curb. Then the traffic light turned from red to green, and he jumped back in his car and drove away. The frame of my wheelchair's small front tire had bent from the heavy impact and only allowed me to get to the mall to use a pay phone for help!

Chapter 28

Society has changed its relationship with disabled people for the better. But in the '70s and '80s, most adults seemed uncomfortable around people with differences. I remember people looking the other way or tugging on their child's arm to hurry away when the child was blatantly staring at me. And most of us with disabilities were treated like we were childlike, regardless of our age. People talked to the person I was with and directed questions meant for me to them—as if I weren't even there—especially in restaurants. The waitress often asked the person I was with what I wanted from the menu. People were much more condescending then than they are now. Not only did I battle with my muscles day in and day out, I also strived to be considered an equal in the public eye. I know I don't have an equal appearance physically, but inside I don't feel different than anyone else.

I truly enjoy being in public places where people treat me equally, open doors with a smile, or offer to get something from a shelf that I cannot reach. Most offer me help without my even asking. The public has definitely improved in its reactions and attitudes towards me since the start of my ordeal. People, especially children, do not stare at me or ask 'What's wrong?' as often as they used to. I believe there are many more people in wheelchairs and other mobility aids out and about in public these days, but it was a much rarer sighting back in the 70's! I'm sure in a movie theatre the people around and behind my seat get distracted by my movement on my bad days, but no one has ever said a thing!

Sometimes I wondered how different life would be without this disorder, but that was a waste of time. It has taken away some independence, including my ability to drive a car, and some everyday choices like wearing high heel shoes. For me, that's just the way it is. One of the bigger annoyances is how dystonia affects my clothing. When I wear full length trousers and slide down in my seat, they ride up to look like I'm wearing capri pants. If I wear capri pants they ride up and in a short time you would think I'm wearing shorts! My tops don't stay in place when my body twists against the back of whatever seat I'm sitting in. Dystonia affects practically everything I do! If I wanted to make light of the situation I would say, dystonia is like a bad circus act that has come into a certain area of my brain but will not pack up its tents and leave!

A Twisted Fate

My childhood and early teen years were my worst years physically in terms of adapting to my malady. But mentally and emotionally, my high school and early adult years were my worst. Although the public's perception of people with disabilities was changing for the better by then, my own perception of myself and others around me made me miserable.

High school at St. Francis Xavier started out fine. I was nervous. It was a big step forward for me. For junior high I went to a school quite far away from my home because of accessibility issues. I had a true, solid friend from the start of grade six until the end of grade nine, but now in high school I was on my own. The school was only a few blocks away from home, and I was still driven to and from school in a cab. Though I did make friends, with an exception or two, they weren't friends after the bell rang to end the school day. My teen social skills were lacking, and though most of my classmates were friendly, they seemed to want to keep a certain distance for the first year or two. I had good friends and good times, but the hard times I went through stood out above all else.

I lost myself for a while. Puberty, self-esteem issues, side effects from medications, and muscles working overtime took their toll. My medications caused drowsiness and made my eyes dry and irritated. At times these side effects drove me wild! I would drift off and be rudely awakened when my head dropped to my chest. Try as I did, I had no control over this. Due to the heavy medications I talked slowly, which may have mistakenly sent signals to people that I was a bit slow mentally. Maybe I was just boring. Who knows? But since I talked a bit slower and was not quick with a comeback, I felt that people were not interested in what I had to say. Then again, that was only my perception at the time!

By now I had a big reclining wheelchair with a raised footrest to accommodate my leg that wouldn't bend. Every moment that I could, I wrapped my left arm behind the left handle of the chair to counteract my twisting to the right. My hip and knee would seldom bend, so I know how awkward I appeared—a big disadvantage for a teen yearning to be equal in an active, able-bodied, high school environment.

I wanted to date. My numerous young crushes and the emotions that romantic novels planted in my head fueled a strong yearning for a relationship. I would always wonder why no male was even trying to make a connection with me, and then I would remind myself that I was in a wheelchair. Who would want to date someone in my condition? Was I embarrassing to be seen with? I thought that more sarcastically than anything else, but on some level it seemed valid. I also felt that dating would make me feel much more equal to others at a time when I felt very self-conscious and far from equal.

High school was also where we learned new things about the world, past and present. I allowed myself to be bothered by a lot of things: seeing others in relationships, global inequality, and the realization that the world was not quite as safe and secure as I thought it was.

The combined effects of the scary world out there, strong medications, slowed speech, low self-esteem, and not having a boyfriend did bad things to my concentration. Slowly my thoughts drifted in and out. Often I could not focus throughout an entire class, so I only had bits and pieces of what I needed to know. If I missed a word or sentence of instruction, I didn't say anything because I thought I would appear stupid. And I would be asking questions all the time. Therefore, I pretended I had gotten the gist of it all.

I wasn't quick with comebacks. I avoided confrontation because I wasn't quick enough to defend myself if need be. The words I needed to properly explain or defend my actions came to me later, but by then it was too late. I didn't believe that my opinion meant much to anyone else anyway, so I just said things that I thought people wanted or expected to hear. I was in a rut not realizing how truly miserable I was. Looking back at entries written in my high school yearbooks, I am reminded of how complimentary and positive my schoolmates were towards me!

I knew the time was coming when I would have to decide what in the world I was going to do with my life. I didn't see any future. Mentally I was not at the top of my game, and I became very introverted in most sur-roundings. I feigned interest and enthusiasm while I par-ticipated in a couple of church youth groups. Although I tried to feel like I belonged among my peers, I didn't. Through the years I always found it easier to converse and get along with adults as opposed to people my own age. Hospital life, especially on an adult ward, meant I was surrounded by adults: doctors, nurses, physical and occupational therapists, roommates, teachers and so on. I did have friends my age, but most of them I found hard to relate to. Their problems were usually quite trivial to me. Everyone has problems, big and small. But other people my age could walk, run, and *be spontaneous.* They had more choices because they were physically independent. It was hard for me to accept. I couldn't enjoy those basics of life.

My mom insisted that I take grade twelve over two years so I wouldn't have such a heavy work load. I dis-liked school so much that I dreaded doing it that way, but I took her advice. The second year was the worst because my classmates from the three years prior were no longer there. I watched in misery as the clock ticked away by the hour, then the minute and then the seconds until I could depart! I did successfully graduate, but not with the grades I should have had. Most of my classmates were excited about their futures. What did mine hold? It was like I was on the outside of life looking in.

Chapter 29

During my second year of grade twelve, 1985-86, Mom and I heard about a neurologist in Vancouver that had some success treating dystonia patients with a drug called Pimizide. I'm sure I could have gotten it in Edmonton, but there were no neurologists here that really knew a lot about dystonia. No neurologist in Edmonton took any real interest in my condition. Instead of following up with me about whether or not the drugs were helping, they just renewed my prescriptions over the phone.

We got an appointment with the doctor in Vancouver at the University of British Columbia (UBC). For the second time, the doctor wanted to admit me on the spot. I broke out in tears. My being admitted was unexpected, so my parents had to go home very shortly afterwards. I spent three weeks in the UBC hospital alone. Thankfully we had some great friends in the Vancouver area who kept in touch with me and whose home I went to on a weekend pass. These friends also lived in Toronto when I was there for my brain surgery.

My head was in the clouds during this time, and I just wasn't noticing a great difference in my movement. Unintentionally, when I talked to my parents over the phone I made my condition sound better than it really was. When I got home, they were eager to see how much better I was doing. It wasn't a big change, and they seemed very disappointed. And so they should have!

Getting in and out of the bathtub was a struggle. Same old story, my left side straightened and my right side was too weak to be of any great help. One day, when I was about fifteen years old, after a bath I leaned awkwardly against the vanity for support and saw my reflection in the mirror. For the first time, something different about my body caught my eye. Simply put, my torso looked crooked. I knew it looked that way because I had a scoliosis due to dystonia symptoms, but I had never seen any physical evidence until that moment. The reflected view of my back told a different story, but how often did I get a good look at my back? Not often. The spine, being close to the surface of the skin, allows curvatures to be seen, but until they're severe they are not easily detected from the front. The deformation of my torso had been slowly happening because of the combined effects of the left side of my pelvis being tugged upward and my progressing scoliosis. I had had a bath a few days earlier and looked in the mirror, but I must have mentally blocked out what I saw. When the denial vanished and I realized what the dystonia was continuing to do to my body, I broke down in a long, deep sob!

Slowly and continuously my movements change and shift. They regress and progress and continually change my body's landscape. That's why I've gone through times of not being able to feed or dress myself, although that is a non-issue at the moment, to being independent enough to live on my own. This twisting and deforming of my body has been a slow and arduous process.

Chapter 30

Once, early in the summer of 1990, I missed a couple doses of medication, which wasn't unusual, but I noticed no difference in muscle activity. It finally occurred to me that I should go as long as I could without medication until I noticed a difference. I didn't detect an increase in movement or discomfort, so I decided to go cold turkey off everything and see how that went. I had a wonderful summer; I was no better, but no worse. To be off medication for the first time since 1974 I was elated, but towards September my movement was once again picking up.

We went to my neurologist-of-the-moment in Edmonton, and he told us a new clinic had opened in Edmonton. It was called the Movement Disorder Clinic and specialized in Parkinson's, Huntington's and dystonia. We were ecstatic because we now had a *specialist* in town. We made an appointment.

Upon meeting Dr. Martin, we sensed he was a gentle, thoughtful man. My mom and I told him about my medical history. He did a quick evaluation of my limbs and left the room. When he came back into the room he declared "Well, you certainly have dystonia." That wasn't exactly what we had come to hear. We were quite aware that that was the case. He said I should go back on medication, which primarily was Artane. That was another thing I hadn't come to hear. Again, I broke out in tears. Artane had irritating side effects that I didn't want to go back to. It caused dry and irritated eyes, dry mouth, and concentration problems. This was the drug that had me done in during high school. So he was quick to suggest Cogentin, or its generic alternative, Benzotropine. It was in the same category as Artane but might not have the same side effects. I jumped at the chance, and it did help to the same extent that Artane did, but without those awful side effects. But just like Artane, Cogentin also produces minimal results.

I have taken medications since day one of being diagnosed. Most of them have been muscle relaxants. I have also taken anti-anxiety meds that are usually prescribed to treat Parkinson's disease or spasticity. After brain surgery I took anti-seizure meds. I've taken some drugs that did me good, but the side effects outweighed the benefits.

Although I am probably forgetting a few, over the years I have taken Haldol, Tegretol, Rivotril, Dilantin, Sinemit, Valium, Dalmane, Artane, Benzatropine, Baclofen, Clonazepam and Ativan (sparingly). The last four are the ones I take now, but I'm not sure how effective they really are. Some days I feel they are doing nothing. I'm not the sharpest knife in the drawer at times, but I truly believe my medications slow me down and bad mental habits acquired in my teens have not completely been disposed of yet. I really want to get off medications because they slow everything down: my reflexes, my speech (to a small degree) and most importantly my energy!

We hear a lot about Botox® these days. It is a diluted form of food poisoning (botulism) that temporarily paralyzes muscles that it comes in contact with. Now it is widely used for cosmetic reasons such as preventing facial wrinkles, but for many years it was used only medically to relieve tightness and spasticity in dystonia and other muscles disorders. The muscles controlling my hip are strong and deep into the tissue. I tried Botox® every three months for one year but did not get any relief. After that the doctor tested my body's response to the drug by giving me injections in my forehead. If after a short time I was not able to move any muscles in my forehead, we would know that it did work for me. If so, my doctor would have to be more accurate at finding my correct muscle group or perhaps use more of the toxin. After getting the shots in my forehead I could still move those muscles, which meant the shots didn't work for me regardless of how accurately the doctor calculated the placement or dosage. Although Botox® didn't work for me, some people get great results until the drug wears off and they have to go back for more. You cannot get these shots more often than every three months to make sure the Botox® has left totally left the system, so if the shots effects wear off in two months you have to wait another month until you get the benefits it provides. Cheers to those it helps!

In addition to taking medications, I have had surgeries, acupuncture, massage, vitamins and the list goes on. If alcohol had ever made even a minimal difference, I would have been an alcoholic years ago, but I'm not!

I'm not really a believer in alternative medicines or treatments. They may work for the common cold or flu, but not for dystonia symptoms. I have tried many of them to no avail. If there is a sure-fire alternative out there I'm sure we will know about it, hopefully sooner than later. This disorder plays hardball and is the toughest of opponents for muscles and anything else that tries to restrain its power.

Chapter 31

I had no idea what I was going to do with my life. The thought of going on to higher education scared the life out of me. With my grades I probably would not have gotten into a post-secondary institution anyway. My concentration was still very poor. My mom levelled with me again. I could take six months off after high school and do nothing if that's what I really wanted, but after that time period I had to have an idea of where I wanted to go and how to get there.

In March of 1987, before I had given a lot of thought to moving out, Rick Hansen wheeled through Edmonton on his 'Man in Motion' world tour. Rick Hansen is of course, Canada's best-known wheelchair athlete. He's well known because of his monumental worldwide tour to raise money and awareness for spinal cord research. He was pushing himself around the world in his wheelchair and was on the last leg of his world tour. Vancouver was where his odyssey started and where it would end.

It was a wintry Sunday, and Rick Hansen was depart-
ing from our city on highway 16 westbound. He was
going to be stopping at the Macdonald's restaurant that
was on his route and near the highway. Since that was on
our end of the city, not all that far away, my mom asked
if I would like to go and hear the quick speech he would
be making outside the fast food restaurant. I thought that
was a great idea, so we jumped in the car to go see him.
When we got there, there were so many cars and people
it was nearly impossible to get close or even get a quick
glimpse of him. Mom then suggested we drive out on the
highway and pull off to the side to wave as he wheeled by.
We were doing just that. Or so I thought.

We parked on the side of the highway, Mom took
my wheelchair out of the trunk, I got in, and then all
we had to do was to wait. There was still snow on the
ground, but it was not too cold out. Soon we could see
him and his entourage approaching and picking up
momentum to conquer the Rocky Mountains and get
home to Vancouver. As they got nearer, my mom all of a
sudden pushed me out into the middle of the highway to
meet him. I was horrified! Here this incredible man was
leaving Edmonton with one and a half provinces to go to
complete his dream, picking up speed and I was going to
interrupt that? They did not come to a complete stop, but
they slowed down, and all I can remember either of us
saying is 'keep on rolling.' That was from him! To make

it more embarrassing, there was a CBC camera crew on the scene. They wanted to interview me on my thoughts of Mr. Hansen and what he meant to me. My mind was a blank, but I did say how impressed I was with him. And when people see him doing extraordinary things like touring the world with only the use of his arms, that reflects on me and what people could expect of me.

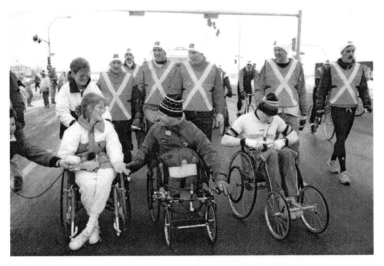

First time meeting Rick Hansen near the end of his Man in Motion Tour. March of 1987.

Later that evening we sat around the TV to watch the news. I was nervous to see myself, assuming I even made it past the cutting room floor. Well I did, but I was not happy. I am extremely grateful for having the gift of speech, but back then whenever I heard my voice on cassette tape I was always shocked and embarrassed because my voice sounded so much deeper and slower than I perceived it to be. That was the case on television too, and I went to my bedroom bawling. I hated how I sounded and even what I said. I was so embarrassed! I was young at that time, but now I know that most people don't like the sound of their voice, and I apologize to those who have real trouble with their speech.

The day before Rick was to arrive back in Vancouver— to much celebration and fanfare—the reporter who interviewed me on that traumatic day not long before called me. She asked if she could come over the next day, watch Rick's live celebration on TV with me, and get my reactions and thoughts throughout the broadcast. I had gotten over the trauma of the earlier interview, so nervously I said yes.

CBC arrived before the broadcast started, and then it was at least an hour until Rick made it to the finish line and cut the yellow ribbon in front of throngs of fans and supporters. I too was a fan and supporter of his efforts. (As the leader of the Dystonia Support Group a few years later, I learned that you have to do extraordinary things to create awareness and get research funds.) But sitting through Rick's arrival, being taped for my reactions, both verbal and facial, was an extremely long and tedious task. The pressure to feel inspired and say something meaningful was strong. What I did say, at my mother's earlier suggestion, was that he had inspired me to think seriously about moving out and becoming more independent. Also, what I thought to be quite cheesy at the time, I exclaimed, "Now I feel like I could climb a mountain!"

In March of 2005, I was lucky enough to meet Rick Hansen under much different circumstances. The setting was a hotel conference room in downtown Edmonton. He was promoting his 'Wheels in Motion' program fundraiser that he was starting up in Vancouver. I was able to talk with him briefly and retell the circumstances of when we met the first time. He of course didn't remember the brief encounter eighteen years earlier, but he laughed and praised my mom for her part.

I had owned and read his book, *Rick Hansen: Man in Motion*, and liked it very much. Among the drama and setbacks he faced on his tour, there were also a lot of humorous stories. I looked high and low for the book to try to get it autographed, but I didn't find it. He told me they were just putting out an updated edition and if I emailed his Vancouver office they would send me a free copy of it. I did that and very quickly had an updated, signed version of *Rick Hansen: Man In Motion*. It was signed 'To Brenda, It was great to see you in Edmonton this March. Never give up on your dreams. Anything is possible! Sincerely, Rick Hansen.'

Inspired and encouraged by Rick Hansen's achievements and message, at the age of twenty I decided that living on my own was what I wanted to accomplish first. I had a disability income and was eligible for a subsidy through the Edmonton Housing Authority. My dad thought I wouldn't be able to function alone and should find a roommate to share the little, adapted two-bedroom townhouse I was renting. My mom thought I would manage fine. She did have some misgivings, but she didn't let on. I was going from an inaccessible home that, due to narrow hallways and doors I could not use my wheelchair in, to an accessible suite in which I could get around very nicely. I was twenty, and it was a cute little place for that stage in my life. The problem was I still wasn't doing anything. Going from school days of getting up early and spending whole days busy in school to a lifestyle of lying around watching TV much of the time, I noticed my unwanted dystonic movement was slowing down!

My confidence and self-esteem have grown over the years, but if I were videotaped for a day and watched the footage I would be mortified and never want to leave the confines of my home. I know I am awkward and deformed to some degree, but that is not how I feel inside my own body. These movements are so normal for me now that I don't think twice about them on a good day, but to visually witness them is a different thing all together. Seeing other people with movement disorders affects me too because I know what they are experiencing and my heart goes out to them. I concluded that I can't let these differences interfere in my life or I will miss out on the things in life that I really enjoy and find fulfilling, even though

A Twisted Fate

I'm still limited! I must not waste energy feeling negative.
If I give off a positive vibe, people respond to that instead
of my differences!

Chapter 32

After I moved out of my parent's home at the age of twenty, I wasn't very motivated to do anything more. What was out there for me? The movement had only decreased a small notch or two, but I was going stir crazy. My mom encouraged me to go to the Rick Hansen Centre, which has since been renamed The Steadward Centre, after its founder, Dr. Bob Steadward. Dr. Steadward's sister Debbie had been my physiotherapist during those crazy cast debacles. Even though I had met both men the centre was named after, I did not have the urge to try it out. Located in the Physical Education Building on the University of Alberta campus in Edmonton, the Steadward Centre is designed for disabled people to work out on their own. The staff assess users' wants and needs and set them up with a personal routine. If anyone needs help at any time, someone is always there to help. My mom urged me on several occasions to try this program out because I was sure to make friends if nothing else.

Finally I made the call, went on a short waiting list and finally went in to be assessed.

I went to this centre three times a week for at least a year. People were really friendly, but adolescence had really been tough so I had very little social confidence and was quite reserved. The exercise routine was a little tough, and I just slowly went through the motions. I wasn't putting out enough energy to do much good, and I tired quickly.

Finally, I decided that work in the travel industry might be something I could be good at and find interesting. I had been lucky enough to travel quite a bit, so I figured I might work exclusively with disabled travelers someday. I enrolled in Travel & Tourism at a private college in a part-time course that ran two nights a week for six months. A good friend was enrolling, so that helped me make my decision. It was really the easy way out, because I could have applied to a higher-quality community college, but I thought it offered the possibility for future employment.

The course was really a waste of time and money. I didn't know much more when I finished than when I started. The majority of things the class offered were videos of popular tourist destinations. The small amount of computer training was obsolete by the time the course was over. Out of ten resumes I sent out to local travel agencies, I got one response.

A Twisted Fate

At my only interview I said I would be willing to work evenings and weekends if necessary. I also said I would like to volunteer for the first few months so I could learn, but I wouldn't be accountable if something went wrong. The owner of the agency had just recently bought the business. I didn't know this at the time. The interview was short because this man didn't know as much about the industry as I assumed he would. I thought he was the expert, and he thought I had more knowledge and experience than I did. So I got the job, and as soon as I made a sale I would be on commission only.

I started by writing every large hotel chain asking for a list of all their properties that had disabled accommodations and to please provide the details and setups of these properties. None of them replied. I could not recommend accommodations to a person with a disability if I didn't know the specifics. I couldn't rely on what reservation clerks or anyone on the other end of the phone would tell me. Most people think that just because they have an elevator in their hotel that they are accessible properties, but that isn't true. Stairs elsewhere in the building, the size and layout of the washrooms, and the amount of open space to move around in the room were other considerations. I had so many questions to ask the other agents, but they needed their time to do their work. I didn't feel comfortable asking questions all the time, but I had to. I did put together a few successful package trips for disabled and non-disabled clients, but mostly I just sold airfare. Being part time is not great for agents in the travel field, and I definitely was not cut out for competition. I was, and to some degree, annoyingly still am, an overly sensitive person in some areas. If I lost a client to someone else it would be crushing and bother me for days on end. My government income did not allow me to make more than approximately $150 a month at the time. I never did exceed that amount, which shows that I wasn't there for the money. I do have to say that the staff members, who came and went very quickly, were wonderful for the most part and I felt they never seemed to view me as 'disabled.'

I did have fun at times. The agency had a big clientele of Spanish people, and therefore, Spanish agents. There was an attractive male agent from Chile who would innocently joke and flirt with me, both of us knowing it was just all in fun. I had never had a flirting experience, and I very much enjoyed the attention. The job was not a total write off for sure, but the travel business was not for me. Finally, due to issues with poor management and more muscle movement, I quit the travel agency.

I regret not having some kind of career, but I know that neither my physical stamina nor my level of concentration could keep up the pace required to get an education and meet the demands of a career. Heidi, my friend from the Glenrose — despite her severe physical limitations — went from the Glenrose School, to part-time enrollment at a mainstream high school and then to the University of Alberta. After nearly eighteen years of part-time studies, she graduated with a Doctor of Philosophy in English! She has written plays that have been featured at the Edmonton Fringe Festival. Her plays are about the guilt that the disabled often feel because they have survived, but some of their friends and class-mates have died early due to their disorders. Her latest play depicts her life and the many traumatic events she has gone through in very thought provoking and original way! She has also written a book based on her thesis. Her research explored the question, 'Should the disabled be out in regular schools if they feel more comfortable staying at a school like the Glenrose?' She also studies issues surrounding euthanasia.

When we talked about her struggle and motivation to accomplish the monumental achievement of getting her Ph.D., she told me people kept telling her she couldn't do it, so she had to prove them wrong. I smiled at that. I told her if I were in that position, people would tell me I *could* do it and I would be the one saying, "No, I can't." I find it interesting but slightly pathetic on my part.

Chapter 33

Dating had always been a sore spot with me. Hindsight is 20/20 isn't it? I wanted someone to ask *me* out because then I would know that they had a true interest in me and were not bothered by my disorder, which can be distracting to say the least. If I asked someone out, I would always wonder what they truly thought of me. If they said yes, were they just being nice to me? Were they trying to humour me? If they turned me down, or had a girlfriend, or for any other reason said no, I could not handle the rejection! I didn't think a girl asking a guy for a date counted as a real date. I did ask a few men to various events, but usually nothing happened. If it did, I was so uneasy and awkward, personifying my disorder, I just wanted to run the other way. I could never get the courage to let the ones I liked the most know my feelings. I thought it would scare them away, so I was left broken-hearted on a few occasions. The feelings were never mutual. I still had little self-esteem.

Shortly after starting at the travel business, I met a man who quickly turned into my boyfriend. I met him at a Christmas social put on by the Rick Hansen Centre. I knew him, but just to say hello. He was also in a wheel-chair. My self-esteem was boosted to a very high level. Someone was finally reinforcing that I was attractive, interesting, and worth the effort to ask out! It was what I needed and wanted to reclaim some self-esteem and belief in myself. It did wonders for me, but for a long time I was on edge believing it might not last long because every other time something seemed to be going my way it was pulled out from under me. But we went together for four years. That was long enough for me to realize that I was okay and content even if I didn't have a man in my life. But I still always wanted one.

A year after breaking up with my first boyfriend, I met a man who would become my husband. My wheelchair and awkward body movements were not an issue with him. He was accepting of my condition from day one. His job exposed him to disabled people every day because he drove for the disabled transportation system I was fairly dependent on. But due to many issues, dystonia not being one of them, we divorced after ten years of marriage.

Most young women start to feel maternal and long to have a family someday, and I was no exception. I thought if I ever did get married, I would consider having one child. But after a while, that feeling faded away. I knew, in the back of my mind, that I didn't want to pass the dystonia gene down the line so, no matter what, I would not have a child. My former husband and I decided this was the right thing to do. I am totally fine now with my decision not to have children. I could not meet the physical demands of a child while trying to meet my own, especially if my child also had dystonia.

I have been blessed with two nieces and two nephews. In 2004 my brother Kevin and his wife Margaret had a darling little girl named Kirsten. They reside in London, England. My sister Trisha is divorced but has three wonderful children. Mandy was born in 1983, Matthew in 1985 and Tyler in 1987. Trisha has since remarried to a man named Gary. Mandy and her husband, Ian, produced Reese, my first great-niece, in 2012! They all reside in Calgary, Alberta.

Some forms of dystonia are hereditary and some are not. In the inherited form, if one parent carries the gene it does not necessarily mean that the parent has any symptoms. However there is a 50/50 chance that the gene will be passed on to offspring. If a child gets the gene, there is only a 30-40% chance the child will develop symptoms. That is a slim window of opportunity. I fit in the window! On top of that, the two complications resulting from my brain surgery, each with only a 2 to 5% chance of happening, happened. Twice! I really should buy more lottery tickets!

I found out years after high school that my father and
grandfather felt twinges of guilt because dystonia had
been passed through their DNA. I felt horrible about
that because they did not know about dystonia or have
any idea they carried the gene. The only other documented case in the family was Rob, and his family had
kept to themselves about the whole thing. And maybe
they weren't aware that it could be passed on. In families with only one or two cases that they know about in
their family history, would everyone give up on having
families? There is a test now—not available in the '70s—
that can detect the gene for generalized dystonia. Some
people want to know and others don't, but it's great to
know that the test is available.

Chapter 34

Getting a job and finding a boyfriend gave me the confidence and the self-esteem I needed. Although it was all overwhelming at the start, I started to take exercise seriously and did mostly cardiovascular activities. My muscles were slightly more agreeable because of my slower lifestyle after high school. I was never overweight, but I trimmed down a bit. Because I had more endurance and confidence I started to develop deep friendships. For seven years I had been going out almost every day, being active, and loving it. I worked twice a week at the travel agency, did physical workouts twice a week, and pursued hobbies such as ceramics class once a week. I had a boyfriend to spend most weekends with doing different activities. But those seven years took their toll, and my dystonic movements, especially in my hip, slowly increased. Regrettably, I had to cut back my schedule.

Taking cues from my muscles, I adjusted my schedule and had to find ways to carry out my daily tasks. I can't eat well on my own if I can't get close enough to the plate, but I cannot be pushed up close to a table because I need room to move around and to push myself back up after my inevitable slide down in my seat. If I'm too closed in, my muscles feel claustrophobic.

I also needed to find a way to sit so I could use my typewriter to do homework and other writing. Without the ability to bend my hip, my options were limited. At school my typewriter was to the right of my desk. I had to twist to the right because I could only type with one or two fingers on my left hand. I was feeding the fire, so to speak, because that was the direction the dystonia was twisting me. At the time it was the only way I could do things, even though I was enabling the twisting motion.

Eating and typing are activities I must do daily. When my hip caused problems, asserting its power by not allowing me to bend forward, I had to find an alternate way to do these things.

Eventually I did. I swung my left leg straight behind me—much like a ballerina, but without the ankle extension and certainly minus the grace and beauty—and kept it there. Or I tucked that leg underneath me and sat on my calf. The latter position gave me the leverage to lean forward and do these types of daily activities. I still have to do things this way on certain days or occasions. I have to sit on the edge of my chair and have enough clearance beside and behind me for my leg to stretch out behind me. It is awkward, and not great for my back and posture, but it's the only way to do what I need to do. It isn't painful, and I block out the awkwardness of it all. It must look like a really bad acrobatic maneuver, but it can be very helpful. Sitting in this position is hard on my muscles and ligaments. I can only sit on my foot and knee for so long when my muscles are overly active before the lactic acid buildup—usually reserved for athletes—begins, and I must abandon the position no matter how much it is helping.

My childhood hobby of making macramé plant holders required that I sit as only a contortionist and I could for a prolonged amount of time. But I enjoyed doing the macramé, and it was a way to earn my own spending money.

My back is another complicated matter that adds to everything else going on. Since my hip insists on straightening and making me slide down in my seat, and my lower torso twists to the right, my back takes a lot of the impact of my unwanted forceful movement. In my early twenties, as the scoliosis in my lower back progressed and my muscles kept twisting, my spine rotated more to the right. So much so, my pelvic bone and ribs were grinding together at times.

This rotation increased the stress at the joints where ribs join the spinal column. Because the vertebrae are stacked one on top of the other, I experienced a popping feeling in my lower left side. It was a lot like popping the bubbles in bubble wrap, personified! It did not hurt, but it was very troubling. The best explanation, without the benefit of an MRI, was that shearing or tearing of ligaments or muscles around the rib/vertebrae joints was taking place. Even so, it wasn't painful.

Although bracing limbs was always problematic, I felt bracing my torso was different because it would aid weakened muscles. After I made several requests, my neurologist consented to having a back brace made for me. The reason I wanted it so badly was that when I was relaxed and sitting nicely in a chair, the left side of my torso acted like a Raggedy Ann doll. With support for my torso, on my good days I could sit fairly comfortably. The first day I wore the brace it seemed to be the answer I was looking for. It wasn't a *cure*, but I was sitting very comfortably and straighter too. But the second time I wore it, my back muscles started a rebellion. Because my torso twisted and curved to the right, a huge amount of pressure from the rest of my back was channeled onto to the weak, lower right side of my back. That pressure produced great strain in that area.

As a result of the stroke, the muscles in the right side of my back were not all that strong. Because of the brace, I lost a lot of muscle tone on the left side of my back also because those muscles weren't being used as much anymore. The right side still gets the strain on a bad day, but I am dependent on the brace when I'm sitting. It can be problematic, but I still feel it was the right thing to do.

Once, at a neighborhood fund raiser, I won a door prize of a gift certificate for a one – hour professional back massage. As you can imagine, I was thrilled. I got on the massage table, but when the woman started the massage my whole body tensed up and was so uncomfortable we couldn't proceed. It ruined all the relief I had been dreaming of. I knew it would have been temporary relief, but still I was disappointed. If my body had been having a good day, a massage would have done wonders—at least for a while. But it didn't work. I was caught on a bad day. With dystonia, there's no way for me to predict what kind of day I'm going to have.

Chapter 35

Dystonia is psychological on some levels, but I think most of it is just me. I often refer to my muscles in the third person. Stubborn beyond explanation, they do have a will of their own. If I start doing something with my mind completely focused on the task at hand, and then I realize how well my muscles are relaxing and cooperating, at that point the affected muscles are alerted. Aware they are being cooperative, which really goes against their nature, they start up again! The first time I tried an adapted bicycle and chair aerobics—two of many activities I've tried to make my body more efficient and active—I felt blessed because of the success and relief I attained. But my muscles caught on to this and fought against me the next time I tried to get the same benefits. Even when I'm at rest, my muscles often clue in. It is uncanny how it works. My mom has learned not to comment if she sees me lying or sitting comfortably because if she says something it may awaken the beast!

I compare this phenomenon to having a bad headache, although I am not comparing the pain, just the process. With a headache, after a while you may take an aspirin and the pain usually subsides. You are naturally going to feel the relief and want to bask in it if only for a while, especially if it is a really bad headache. Well, very little conscious basking goes on in my mind and body if I find something that gives relief! My dystonic muscles can't bear to see me repeat anything that offers relaxation and comfort on a conscious level. Because of this aspect of the disorder, many people that try to get disability insurance run into problems. The insurer will argue, 'Well, if you can do a certain job one day, then why not the next?' And there is no concrete explanation to give!

When my mom or dad observed me sitting in an awkward position, they often commented on it. Wouldn't I be more comfortable if...? But strangely enough, the awkward position was usually more comfortable and relaxing than a normal position. Most of the time I've felt like a square peg trying to fit in a round hole! It's strange that my muscles cannot function and relax in the normal way. Regardless of where I am, if my left knee is bent and my foot is resting on the floor, sometimes when a person is passing by me my leg will lift up. This reflex often results in my tripping or kicking the person who has entered my personal space. Try explaining that to the unsuspecting victim!

Chapter 36

I have a high threshold for discomfort and certain types of pain. It is something that has evolved out of necessity. I have total sensitivity in my legs, but I will often have scrapes, shallow cuts, or bruises on my legs and have no idea when or where I got them. They happen from the clumsiness of moving around. It took years to become somewhat desensitized to my movement, but I guess the brain does that for you while you struggle through it all. I am just referring to my general movement. On bad days, the movement becomes the focus of my thoughts. Merely thinking of doing an activity will stir up quieted muscles at those times!

Most individuals with dystonia experience on-going pain. That is not the case with me, but it's easy enough to understand why it would be painful. Muscles tighten and pull to the point they twist bones that create permanent, unnatural postures. Most times the movements and twisting are unrelenting. My muscles still turn against me, but I think the reason I don't experience chronic pain is that I wage an intense campaign of counteracting the pull of my muscles by pulling them in the opposite direction when possible. I am incredibly flexible on my left side, although my ligaments have probably been stretched to their limits. Ligaments are like strong elastics holding bones together, but if they're stretched too much they do not recoil. If I let the muscles do what they wanted without a battle, I wouldn't have the movement and range of motion I do. My affected muscles would be more rigid and unrelenting. So movement is my problem, and now, partly my solution. My commitment to fighting back with opposing movement *seems* to be helping. I must keep moving so I don't stiffen up completely.

Everyone with dystonia has to do whatever works for them. I have my own theories, but I would never advise someone to do things my way just because it works for me. If you can stretch a muscle group without exacerbating the current problem or creating other problems, I feel it's a must do! If I had torticollis, (dystonia in the neck) yanking my neck in the other direction may not be possible or safe to do. I think it is instinct that you clearly draw upon! I am incredibly concerned about experiencing pain in the future, but I am preparing myself as best I can to minimize its strength. My body has been extremely resilient!

While living with dystonia, you will often find a relief mechanism. This means that you can find a position or a certain movement that will allow a symptom to cease, although the sense of relief is fleeting. In my case, it is to elevate my straight left leg and rest it on an object about the height at which I am sitting or higher. This sometimes relieves negative muscle movement in my hip. A lot of variables have to be considered, such as seat height and the height and solidity of the other object. If I can wedge my foot tightly between my chair and the object, that is all the better for short, but welcome, relief. And of course, my muscles have to be in the mood too! I try to overshoot my target, whatever it might be, so it is easier to achieve it.

I have come across a few other comfortable positions through the years, but they lose their effectiveness I use them too often. My most relaxing position, when I'm ready to sleep, is the last of a series of stretches that must take place before I lie on my left side in bed. I leave the best until last. In a similar vein, at meal time I eat the food I least enjoy first and then eat the food I really like last. That way I end the meal feeling satisfied. It helps develop tolerance. If I ride a situation out for a while, I may have a better ending. If I take the most effective route to relaxing, it seems only a matter of time until its effectiveness wears off. It's partly how I have managed to tune out many of the bothersome things going on in my body; that is, not doing the first or only action for relief. My brain can catch on to these types of things. In the past, my body would catch on to something that was helpful to me, only to dry up what amounts to be my oasis in a desert.

Chapter 37

There is a lot of variation among people with dystonia regarding their symptoms and the effectiveness of various treatments. I've been telling **my story**, but there are individuals with different forms of this disorder whose stories have not been made public. (There is a list of dystonia and the forms it can take at the conclusion of this book.) Here are three personal stories from individuals I have known personally, or have knowledge of. These brief, condensed accounts of their daily struggles with different forms of dystonia touch on how it has changed their lives dramatically.

- A lady named Lou searched twelve years for answers before a doctor finally diagnosed her with **spasmodic dysphonia (dystonia that affects vocal cords)**. She had seen many speech therapists who gave her suggestions to help her cope with her speech problems. One therapist was less than helpful during a session that was not going well. She boorishly suggested that Lou repeat what she said in the same way she, the therapist, was speaking. Her voice was stern, like she was scolding a stubborn child. Lou proclaimed 'If I could speak like you, I wouldn't need a therapist or treatment, now would I?' Stating that she would never be back, Lou left the room and reported the therapist to her employer. She went to every specialty doctor she could and when she finally realized she had never seen a neurologist for this condition, she went to one and fortunately got the correct diagnosis. At that particular appointment, the neurologist was taken aback when she jumped off the examining table and gave him a gratitude-induced bear hug. For twelve years her voice had been deteriorating—sounding deep, forced, and breathy. Many people thought she just had a cold that wouldn't go away. She was also terrorized while sleeping. She will wake up with the sensation that she is being strangled, fighting to breathe as though someone's hands were gripping her throat. Eating is not a problem, but when she drinks something, aspiration often occurs. She is helped by Botox® injections every three months. They cannot be given any more often than every three months because the toxin needs time to totally leave the system.

- Susan contracted **oromandibular dystonia**, which affects the jaw, face, and/or the tongue. The first

symptoms she had showed up when she was eating something. Without warning, her jaw would
snap shut and cause severe, painful wounds to her
tongue. The time came when her jaw was clenched
shut at all times. The muscles on the side of her
face were painfully strained. Sometimes before
trying to sleep, as a relief mechanism she would
attempt to wedge a fingertip between her upper
and lower teeth just to take the edge off the clenching. The worst problem was she could not eat, so
she could only drink liquids through a straw! To
walk through a mall and have to pass a food court
was too much to bear because of the smell of all
her favourite foods that she could no longer eat!

- Bill had some mild psychiatric problems and sought
treatment. Doctors put him on medication in hopes
of treating his problems. Some medications used
to treat mental health concerns can cause dystonic
symptoms. That's what happened with Bill. He
started developing **secondary dystonia** and was
having a terrible time with uncontrollable muscles
in many regions of his body. He didn't know where
to turn for help regarding the unwanted movement,
and his doctors continued to prescribe the same
medications to treat Bill's psychiatric problems.
He later learned that if people stop taking the
medications soon after the dystonic symptoms

appear, the movement problems usually go away. But if people are kept on these drugs for a prolonged period of time, the dystonic symptoms will stay. His doctors would not take responsibility for this oversight. Some doctors say that if the dystonia stays under these circumstances, it was there all along. But the symptoms might not have been triggered had he not been given those drugs for a prolonged period of time!

A common experience is the lengthy process of getting diagnosed. After that, finding helpful information about how to deal with the disorder is a challenge. Cancer, diabetes, multiple sclerosis, arthritis, spinal cord and brain injuries are all terrible disorders and well deserving of the same things: research, donations, awareness, and patient support. But the difference is, if you stop a person on the street, or a medical professional in a hospital, and ask them if they have heard of the above mentioned disorders, you will most likely get a yes. Ask the same people if they have heard of dystonia and chances are they will say no. You are not likely to donate to a cause you have never heard of or know nothing about. Also, you will not be able to tell a friend or family member that is suffering with a nagging, twisting limb or body part that the problem may not be "all in their head." It is quite common for a person with dystonic symptoms to hear a friend say 'I saw a blurb on the news' or 'I saw a short article in the paper, and it sounds like you might have a thing called dystonia.' From there they get themselves referred to a neurologist who will hopefully give them a correct diagnosis.

Now we can thank the internet for helping us find information much quicker, but in the early 1970's Sam Belzberg, a Canadian businessman, was frustrated when his young daughter was diagnosed with generalized dystonia. The family had many questions but very few answers about dystonia and what could they do about it. He gathered up all the resources he could find and created the Dystonia Medical Research Foundation (DMRF) in 1975. The foundation has three goals: to raise awareness, to support the diagnosed, and to fund research. A lot of work went into getting it up and running, but once established the momentum grew and it is a wonderful foundation with its three goals firmly in place. It provides information in the form of pamphlets, newsletters, DVDs and so on. It hosts symposiums for patients and medical personnel together. The DMRF has children's groups and special interest groups such as Musicians with Dystonia. Support groups have been established in major cities and are now sprouting up in smaller communities too. The foundation supports group leaders and individuals in any way it can. Its staff suggests activities but leaves it up to each support group to decide what they want to do.

The foundation funds grants for researchers who are studying a specific aspect of the disorder. Every year the word about available grants is getting out to more researchers. Sometimes the requests for grants exceed the amount of money DMRF is able to give.

Public awareness about dystonia and the DMRF is crucial for raising research funds.

The Dystonia Medical Research Foundation started in Canada, but now its headquarters is in Chicago. The Canadian chapter, based in Toronto, has a strong working relationship with the Chicago office. There are dystonia foundations in other countries also.

In the early 1990s, a few people who had some form of dystonia banded together to find others with it in the Edmonton area. My parents and I were located and asked to get together to meet, talk, and share our experiences as others would share theirs. With some hesitation on my part, we attended this meeting. Approximately twelve people, including some who brought family members for moral support, were present. One fellow had developed pulling and twisting of his neck after suffering whiplash in a bus accident. The others did not know how their dystonia originated. One woman had segmental dystonia which affects a limb and an adjoining body part. This woman had it in her neck and shoulders. Parents of a girl who was barely into her teens talked about her struggle with generalized dystonia and how it took eight years to get a correct diagnosis. At times the room was full of anger and frustration because of the difficulties people had gone through up to that point. Some had gone years without doctors having any answers for them.

This disorder, at least until properly diagnosed, is very alienating. Your muscles pull or twist whatever body part dystonia is affecting in odd and erratic ways, and no one can give you an answer as to why. Many have been told that it is just a bad case of stress and "it's all in your mind." Or you or your loved one is just seeking attention, which I know is infuriating because I had that particular judgment handed down on me. After being told these things repeatedly, some people believe it and withdraw, left wondering how something as strange and often painful can be caused by something they have done to themselves. Perhaps there are some attention-seekers out there; I can't say for sure. But if a doctor tells you "it's all in your head" and you disagree, get a second, third, fourth or fifth opinion. Doctors can't know everything, but some just won't admit that they don't! Most victims just find relief knowing what they have is real and has a name!

People alienate themselves from family, friends and life because it is just too much to deal with: the loss of control, extreme pain, and *no answers!* Everyone at this meeting had a horror story, and they really needed to meet others they could relate to and understand.

Eventually a local support group was put together where people could share stories about the kind of hell they went through until their child or relative was finally diagnosed with dystonia. The group was also a place to share information and get some answers. I shied away from getting too involved in the group. After being so alienated from others with this muscle-seizing disease, it was mentally difficult for me to see others with uncontrollable muscles at that point in time. I knew deep inside that I should get more involved, but I really didn't want to.

Edmonton and its surrounding area truly needed a support group. I had had this disorder for approximately seventeen years at the time, and I knew of only two or three cases in Edmonton. But it was more a case of knowing *of* them, not *knowing them*. My Mom could have used that support when I was diagnosed. A support group was established. We elected a president to help us grow and promote awareness of dystonia. She was the mother of the young teen with the severe case of generalized dystonia. She was very motivated and did a good job. Under her direction we organized a gathering with a pharmaceutical company to inform people about what their medications could possibly do for them. We also hosted a regional symposium that brought in medical specialists from other regions of Canada to be the speakers. The Foundation provided financial help for this event. Our group did a few fundraising activities too.

To increase awareness about dystonia we put together information packets for doctors, and we dropped them off at clinics around the city. Some members reported that at certain clinics the receptionist or head nurse was less than enthusiastic about these packets, so we were never sure whether the doctors ever saw them or not. All we could do was try. If the doctors were to read through this info, they would be closer to knowing about us and possibly want to know more.

After a couple years of leading this group, the president announced she was giving up her role as leader. If no one else was willing to take the position of president, the group would cease to exist. I knew that this group was essential to our city and region, but I had never been a president of anything before so I never even considered the option. Me? Be the president of a support group that represented not only Edmonton but all of Northern Alberta? But my mom spoke up to volunteer me and another girl, Janice, mentioned earlier, who also had generalized dystonia, to share the job as co-presidents. There was hesitation on both our parts but we finally agreed. The group could not fold!

After only a year of sharing the duties, my co-president found a teaching job outside of the city and left for a new challenge. I was now *the* president. My standard duties were writing a newsletter at least three times a year and holding meetings. I was a very informal leader.

I didn't have minutes taken with old news and new news and so on. My newsletter covered all that.

It was a difficult task to get members to participate and share. As much as I wanted to, I could not chastise members for not participating, but it was hard to keep hinting that these meetings were for their good, not just mine! The purpose of the meetings was to listen, or join in the discussion, and share stories of ordeals or things that have been helpful. They could bring friends and family to enlighten them about what they were going through, and in doing so perhaps help others. Occasionally I invited a guest speaker, but I felt sharing and opening up would be good for the soul and encourage friendship building. I knew there was much more I could be doing, but I did what I could handle which is all anyone was required to do. I definitely didn't want to bite off more than I could chew. Every once in a while, when a member mailed in the nominal membership fee they included a short note praising me for doing a good job. Thank you!

Lou, the woman described earlier with spasmodic dysphonia, met my mom at church. When she heard Lou's forced, husky speech, on a hunch, my mom asked her if she had dystonia. She looked at my mom with disbelief. It was a week after she had been diagnosed! She then learned that there was a support group in our city and couldn't have been happier or more grateful to find this out and get at least *some* of the help and information she was looking for!

After twelve years of leading the group, I realized it was time for a change. I had a challenging yet fulfilling time being president.

The Dystonia Medical Research Foundation is terrific. Support groups can do as little or as much as they want. There are no guidelines to follow unless you ask for them. And when you ask, you get them! Every year the foundation encouraged each group to hold a Run, Walk & Wheel event as a fundraiser. For a few years I declined holding one in our city because of the workload involved. The task list provided by the DMRF included obtaining the required permits, getting paramedics to volunteer their time, taking care of registrations, and many other jobs. The list was helpful, but organizing the event was a lot of work for one person. Although I had a few people that would help, it still seemed like too much work to take on.

I was not the most original or lucrative fundraiser, but I coordinated a hot dog sale at a local grocery store. The average amount raised per year was $300, and I would ship it off to the Canadian office for research dollars.

Then one day I got a phone call from a woman whose son had been diagnosed a few years earlier with generalized dystonia. I had heard about Connie and her son. Her best friend had contacted me at an earlier date telling me about the struggle her family was dealing with. I knew that someday, when she and her family felt better adjusted to this devastating intrusion that her teenage son was facing, she would give me a call.

Connie knew about the Foundation and asked if I had ever held a Walk, Run &Wheel fundraiser before. When I told her I hadn't, she asked if we could hold one if she took on the head role of planning the activity. I said, 'Yes, by all means. That would be wonderful.' With great help from a small group of people, Connie and I pulled off a stunning success. By getting her son's school, their family synagogue, and friends involved with all the other participating members' families, we truly amazed ourselves by having over 300 people come out. We raised over $16,000! We were able to keep up that momentum for two more years before we showed signs of burnout. Connie's organizational skills formed a template for all of Canada's groups to follow if they choose to.

In place of Walk, Run & Wheel events we do a letter-writing campaign that has been just as successful financially. Members send a form letter to people they know who might be willing to give a donation. Sam Belzberg, DMRF founder and a successful business man, held golf tournaments in our area, and for three years our group was the beneficiary of the proceeds. Now we get partial proceeds from working Alberta Gaming and Liquor Commission casinos. As of August, 2012, we have raised over $550,000 for research!

Chapter 38

All the emotional ups and downs, the surgeries, and of course the effects of dystonia, have made me who I am today. My body has shown great resilience, but it also shows the evidence of my long battle with the unwelcome intruder. I have many surgical scars as well as two indentations in my skull. Each body part that has been commandeered has its unique set of problems and limitations. My left foot is usually clenched within an inch of its life. It often scrunches up and acts like one big knot of solid muscle and bone. My two biggest left toes cross, and the other three curl under. My left knee and hip fight to remain extended, my torso curves and twists to the right. My lower legs have an anorexic-like appearance. My right arm is bent across my upper body, and my fist is still tightly clenched but not as bad as before the stroke. My left leg is shorter than the other. My belly button does not line up with other body parts the way it once did. My left arm has tremor and fine coordination issues. My left rib cage juts out when I attempt to lie flat. And of course, I have a scoliosis.

I must clarify that I do not have *constant* movement every day, and when I do it may not last all day! I can walk a few steps at a time but only when I have a steady object to grasp when I get to my destination. Often I just land on my knees after a few steps if I don't feel confident that I will make it. Then I awkwardly crawl to my destination, but usually not when others are around.

I live independently but with a lot of great support. Despite my disorder, I can do a lot more than most people realize. Dystonia usually creates a tug-of-war effect in opposing muscle groups, such as the groups responsible for bending or straightening a leg. But some of my muscles work normally. For example, my left knee will always fight me if I try to bend it, but I can use my left leg and knee, with normal function and strength, to go from a kneeling to a standing position. This is why I'm capable of doing some things that most people wouldn't think I could do!

I'm determined to do as much as I can on my own. I don't know if I've done the right things for my body or any other area of my life, but my decisions felt like the best thing at the time. I realize that pushing too hard and taking shortcuts are actions I profess to be working hard to avoid, but I still do some of them because I want to! I'm very stubborn, but not in the right way. I guess it is still a matter of denial. The stakes get higher as I age. I must lose my stubborn ways and always do what is in the best interest of my body.

No one knows what the future has in store for them, and I am no exception. Sometimes when my thoughts turn to the future and what *might* happen physically, a little hand seems to take hold of my heart muscle and gives it a quick, terrifying yank. At these most intense times my future looks very bleak. But I also know that it might not be bad after all. Anything can happen! Although dystonia is progressive, it helps to know it can regress in some instances.

Finding a way to rid the world of this diabolical intruder called dystonia is up to medical scientists. For my part, I try to give back to all the people whose efforts helped me live a better life, and I hope to be of help to others who are dealing with the disorder. I hope this book will raise awareness, and if I help one person it will be worth it. But most of all, I pray that research leads to a cure for this bizarre affliction. One important reminder is that the symptoms, and my body's ability to respond to them, depend on surroundings and circumstances. There is always an exception to every rule regarding dystonia symptoms.

In this book I have tried to describe what it is like to live with dystonia, and I believe I have more than scratched the surface. But there is a great deal more to living with this disorder that only other people living with it could describe and relate to! For the most part, my life is unfolding the way I want it to. But it will never be exactly how I want it. I have to bend my life around other people's schedules. This isn't fair or easy sometimes, but that's the way it is. The number of hours I have waited for doctors, for other health professionals, and for transportation is beyond measure. Wait times for doctors and other health professionals have become somewhat shorter over the years, but wait times for disabled transportation have not. I am extremely time oriented. The amount of time I have spent waiting borders on the absurd and ridiculous. My time is not my own! I try to be thick skinned about it, but it is still terribly hard to deal with. It is getting harder to deal with rather than easier as time goes on. Independence is crucial and so desired because a lot of time has been taken away and wasted; time I will never get back!

As frustrating as this is, I still try to focus on the positives in my life.

Chapter 39

When I decided to write this book I didn't realize the monumental task I was taking on. To go back in time and recall how it all started and how rapidly this movement disorder progressed was not easy—mentally, emotionally or physically. But within this personal story, I've tried to let you know how much power these muscles have and how truly awkward and frustrating life has been since the summer of 1974! Because of the complexity of the body and the brain, adequately describing what it feels like *internally* is beyond my writing ability. On any given day since that summer my muscles have either been tugging, tensing, twisting, or wreaking havoc in one body part or another.

But I do get good days where unwanted movement is minimal. On a good day, I can sit fairly still and life is generally quite manageable. On a bad day, muscle tensing and twisting intensifies so much that I wonder if I have any future beyond my front door! But, my body is still very resilient!

Struggling with dystonia is a part of my daily life. It has never been easy, nor has the intruder shown any signs of leaving. Since I am used to living with dystonia, sometimes it feels normal; that is, until I sit down and think about it! After going through the process of recalling everything that has happened, I conclude: What a bizarre disorder! Dystonia is like a computer hacker that can tap into a seemingly secure device and spread viruses that ruin its system. It doesn't ruin its ability to function, but it screws up the entire operating system. It's so elusive that it's hard to diagnose and impossible to delete. This hacker has given new meaning to some old expressions:

Change is constant. *I don't like change, but it is happening all the time.* Things can turn quickly from good to bad and from bad to good. This disorder cannot and should not be underestimated, which I myself tend to do when I'm having a good day. On a bad day even shifting my position or moving a limb can be enough to start my muscles contracting. I often try to predict how I will feel the next day based on how I feel in the evening. I'm wrong nine times out of ten! Usually it's not as bad as I thought it would be.

My mom got frustrated to no end whenever we went to see a doctor to try to get some symptoms under control. She would describe the symptoms I'd been having, and I'd be sitting there nice and peaceful. Mom would beg me to start showing the doctor what she meant. She would emphasize that the muscle movements and changes in posture really did happen, but she wasn't really sure the doctor understood or believed her. She would end up doing her own re-enactments! That is truly the nature of this disorder. Some symptoms can come and go on a daily, weekly, or monthly basis and can do so even at the most inopportune times, such as a doctor's appointment. At this point there are so many body parts affected, each with its own strange movements and needs, that I cannot establish a pattern for predictability to save my life. My coordination sometimes seems non-existent, because each part of my body is doing its own thing.

Another unwelcome reality is that once I get a problem solved or under control, another one is just waiting in line to replace it! I have to acknowledge that, rather than try hopelessly to avoid it! I adapt for as long as I can to my surroundings. It's natural now. Instinctively, I am always on the counter attack, always fighting back in order to slow or stop movement, tightness, and eventual posture change. Some movements are visible to the naked eye and some are not. It would surprise some people to know that many movements are not caused by dystonia; they are a deliberate and conscious attempt on my part to counteract the dystonic movement.

Life is full of tough decisions. When I was a child, my parents had to make some difficult decisions regarding surgeries, medications, schooling and so on. You may wonder why, after all these surgeries, most of which caused permanent or temporary side effects, did my parents keep on agreeing to these procedures on my behalf? My mom, after seeing so many children with different disabilities who, short of a miracle, had little hope of regaining their independence, knew that dystonia has a rare distinction: partial reversal of symptoms is possible, and in rare cases, almost full reversal may occur. Although these reversals of fortune are usually not permanent, any one of the many procedures I tried *could have* turned things around dramatically.

But there are some decisions only I can make, and I am given many choices to make in a day. Everyone is. Some are simple, some are not! One decision for me may be this: If I'm feeling well rested on the couch, shall I stay there most of the day or risk losing the well-rested feeling to get up and do things I need or want to do? They have equal importance, and I can go either way. Resting wins most of the time, but getting up to do things I want to do helps me to gain endurance and mental exercise. Sometimes I have to accept the position I'm in and sometimes not.

One of the most frustrating things about living with this disorder happens when I find a comfortable position or activity. I realize that my body is resting or doing something fairly normal, and that realization triggers a muscle rebellion. It is like waking a beast, and it's impossible to ignore! I don't know how I can direct my thoughts away from muscles that are demanding my attention. I could have much better days if I could carry on without my body and mind clashing as they tend to do. Worse yet, I end up feeling guilty about sabotaging my own comfort even though it is not a conscious decision on my part.

On the bad days I face many dilemmas. Do I keep my back in as proper a position as I can achieve but let my foot, knee and hip pull and tug at their own will? Do I overuse my left arm and hand to tug my toes up from their clenched tight position for some temporary relief? Do I drug myself up (with prescribed meds) and hope the tenseness and movement subside just a bit knowing my concentration and mental energy will subside as well? Do I continue wearing the back brace to sit straight on a day that my movements strain the right side of my back or irritate the skin under my arms? It is extremely hard to know what's right or wrong!

Necessity is the mother of invention.

Owning a home has made me learn to do some things out of necessity. I really surprise myself with the things I can do, even though I usually do these tasks in an unconventional way and at a slower pace than normal. Although I'm a perfectionist at heart, I have come to terms with the fact that I can't always do these tasks to my standards. For example, I can wrap gifts, clean up the multitude of spills and messes I make (mostly in the kitchen) and do some light gardening. At times I doubted I would ever be doing things like this. This doesn't mean that my disorder has subsided greatly—the symptoms and challenges are still there—but I am better equipped to deal with things. Time brings wisdom and experience. Actually I would like to get more accomplished in a day. Sometimes my body will let me know it's time to stop, sometimes I will not be aware until it's too late!

I yearn to get up and do the things that might involve overdoing it, but I have to think of what my body needs more. Finding a happy medium is what I need to do, but it is unlikely to happen given the circus atmosphere in a certain area of my brain! And I must admit I'm good at hearing my instincts, but I don't always follow them or put them into practice.

For example, I am prone to taking short cuts or tuning out discomfort as best I can. I forget that I can often find other ways to cope that have less negative impact on my body. I have learned never to do something the same way twice! That way, I hope to avoid the risk of falling into more bad habits and perhaps starting up new repetitive patterns. I find inventive ways of doing things, but I feel any personal example of mine won't make sense to most people. There are many different ways of doing tasks, ways that others would never think about doing only because they haven't had to. I'm sure most people have heard about people with no arms that learn to do everything with their feet. Well, that's the best relatable comparison I can make. I'm still learning after all of this time that if I think way outside of the box, I can find different, unconventional ways of doing things that I'd never thought of before in order to keep going.

I still have to remind myself that there are things I can do to help the situation I'm in. My desire to do an activity quickly to get it over and done with is usually just a bad habit, and I could possibly rethink the task and do it differently. I realize there is no figurative or literal fire. I should do a task with a plan in mind; for example, if I get into my wheelchair to go from the front room to the kitchen, I usually do not sit as straight as I can. I just sit awkwardly because it will not be a long commute, but if I took the time and effort to sit straight each time, it may help more than I know! But as I have mentioned, I usually just want to get a task over and done with before taking these helpful hints seriously! If I can avoid having to directly deal with my muscles, I will sometimes take that option.

Sometimes you just have to let off some steam. People tell me how well I do with the challenges I've had to face. But really, I get by on the fact that I didn't have a choice in acquiring this disorder. I just try to find my way around as best I can. Stress can take a big toll on people, especially those with dystonia. That certainly pertains to me. I handle stress well, all things considered. But it does build up slowly and the smallest issue can set me off! I have three main ways of purging my pent up emotions.

Humour is a must have in my life! I love humour, and I love to laugh. My sense of humour is a little off beat though. I will often laugh at small, quirky things that others don't find funny, and I find humour in some tense or bad situations. I can recall things I've laughed at in the distant past, and I'm still able to laugh and remember the reason for it. It must be the endorphins that laughing releases into the blood stream that cut stress. If I didn't laugh, I would probably cry.

One day in fifth grade, my friend Heidi and I started laughing at some little thing, and it ballooned and we couldn't stop. The laughing lasted most of the day, and by the end of the school day our somewhat strict teacher was quite upset with us. She gave us a killer glare when the laughter started up again. Ever since then, I sometimes laugh at tense moments out of nervousness or uncertainty. I really believe that humour helps me cope, and it definitely lowers stress. *I like the lighter side of life and laugh at silly things, but I can handle the tougher sides of life also. I have been there!*

My second stress reliever is **giving in**. Struggling with uncontrolled movement and twisting, day in and day out, gets extremely old and tiring. I try to be proactive by keeping flexible; otherwise, my muscles will gain more strength and tighten that much more. But there comes a breaking point. I give in! If this intruder wants control, then who am I to stop it? I can't! Why try? Is it ever going to stop? If it wants me to twist, tug, pull, spasm, tense up, slide down in my seat and deform me even more, then bring it on! There comes a time when I'll give in to those muscles just for a little peace of mind. If and when I do that I give away power, but at that point in time I no longer care. It's comparable to a bad police interrogation. The cops will try to break you down until you confess to a crime you didn't even commit just so they'll leave you alone! Thankfully I don't feel forced to give in often, and I don't stay in that frame of mind for long. On the other hand, I will often give up a comfortable twisted position because the temporary comfort comes at the expense of my posture. I'll never figure out why being twisted into terrible posture is more comfortable than sitting and holding a normal position!

My last-resort stress relieving technique is the **melt down**. *Although it does not happen often*, the stress, frustration, and anxiety in my life will hit the boiling point. I have learned to take stress and frustration quite well, but occasionally it builds up to a point where I've had enough! In the privacy of my own home I will get violent and stupid. I will scream until I'm hoarse and in tears, yell ridiculous allegations into the air, and occasionally throw things. Most times I have just enough self-control to know how stupid it would be to destroy certain objects. I do not do this with anyone present! This is one source of stress relief that is best avoided when possible, but it can be very cleansing. And then I move on!

Patience is a virtue. I've been told I had extreme patience when I was younger, but the waiting I've had to endure since then has multiplied by thousands. Out of pure necessity; that is, to keep my sanity, I have learned to adapt and accept the reality of waiting. But the longest and most obvious wait is for my dystonic muscles to surrender. So the wait goes on. The best reward for all this patience would be a cure for dystonia in all its forms.

The squeaky wheel gets the oil. Mom has been my mom, my friend, my disciplinarian, and my tireless *advocate* for things I needed and deserved much before *I* knew I needed or deserved them. An advocate is what every patient needs within the medical system. If my mom hadn't gone out of her way and stuck up for me, I would not be where I am today. Not only would I not be where I am because of her advocacy, but I wouldn't have learned that skill for myself. It took a while to learn how to stand up for what is best for me and to feel comfortable doing so. I'm still learning, but I can do it. The Dystonia Medical Research Foundation and the DMRF Canada are also good resources for advocacy and networking with other families. Other countries have similar organizations for people with dystonia.

Mom has also tried to help medical professionals. She went in search of medical researchers that were working on dystonia. It was hard to track them down since very little was going on, but when she got a clue as to where this might be happening she offered my involvement and/or medical records to help them in their endeavors.

You don't have to go it alone. All my family and friends have helped in many different ways, and I thank them all very much. But my mom truly stands at the front of the line. She has never had an easy life, but you'd never know it by her spirit! Her childhood was traumatic, so she drew on her faith to get her through. God works in mysterious ways. Oddly enough, when my mother was a child, her parents would drop her off at Sunday school, but they didn't stay to attend church themselves! I think God knew she would need extra faith and strength in her future.

My mom and I have our differences at times, but the disagreements don't last long and we carry on. We think differently but have similar goals. My entire family has gone through this with me, but Mom has amazing depth of character. I don't know where her instincts to do the right thing came from, but I thank God for her! We went through a lot together, often without my dad and siblings nearby. I think they understand that this wasn't a choice, and my mother had to take more time with me. It was a sacrifice of great proportions on her part. Dystonia came without directions! We did what had to be done.

She has never let me down. She gave me the kicks I needed at the right time and never treated me any differently in the mothering way. On top of her responsibilities as a mother, a wife, and my caregiver, she always had a part-time job to make sure her children were able to have a few extras in life. If my mom hadn't worked, things like piano lessons, skiing, family trips and more, never would have happened. She pulls her weight but does not tolerate too much drama or foolishness. I don't know how she does it!

She wanted to say a few words about our lives' ups and downs. I think she's earned the right! Here they are:

Dear Brenda,

As your mother, I am so proud of you. I have really been blessed to have you as a daughter. The years passed by so quickly. There have been so many emotions over the years.

In the early stages of your disease there were so many setbacks and struggles. At the time they just seemed to be too much for us all to take in. But we could only take it one step at a time and carry on. It was very hard for your dad and me to see you suffer so much, but you always seemed to have a smile on your face even when things were not going very well. Never once did you say "WHY ME?" You were truly blessed to be able to accept everything that has happened to you.

I always would tell people you never accept your child having a very debilitating disease, you just learn to live with it. But you just seem to be able to get on with the next step in your life. I still marvel at your strength. We know that you struggle with daily tasks that we take for granted.

The last few years we have watched you grow into a lovely young woman.

You have helped many people over the years who also suffer from dystonia. You are able to give them information and can give them first-hand advice and encouragement. You have the ability to show people that there is NO MOUNTAIN TOO HIGH.

Brenda, we know that each day has its struggles for you, but we will be there for you whenever we can.

WE LOVE YOU AND GOD BLESS YOU THROUGH THE MANY YEARS AHEAD!

Love Mom

Throughout my years of struggle, my parents have always supported and encouraged me to follow opportunities as they came along. In between all the major events of my past, I've also lived large. Among all these events that have taken me down such a weird, sometimes dark alley, there has been a lot of light in other areas. I have travelled quite a bit and made many friends. The excitement and wonderful occurrences, despite everything that happened as a child, were not lost on me. They at least partially compensate for all the trouble I've gone through.

My family is not perfect, and there have been a lot of big bumps in the road, but we have managed to stay close despite my siblings' moving away from Edmonton. It is rare for us all to be together at the same time, but it happens every once in a while! We have had some very tense, emotional crises in our family through the years. I tend to downplay the effects dystonia has on my life when I'm having a good day, but it has been an extremely rough ride not only for me but those close to me. My family has had very turbulent moments when we could have cracked right down the middle!

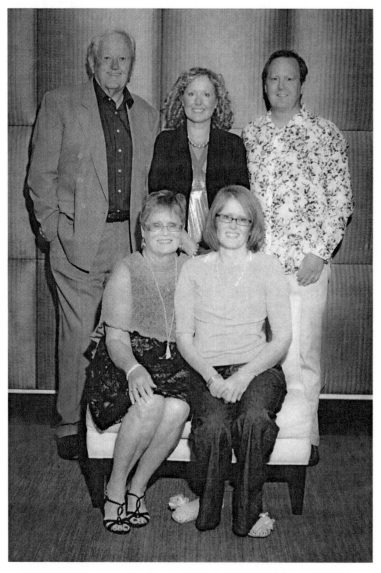

*Here we are 45 years after our first family photo! This was
taken on Mom and Dad's 50th Anniversary! August 2011.*

I truly thank my family for their support and unwavering efforts to keep me and my life as normal as possible. I have not been treated any differently than my siblings. I got in as much trouble as they did. Any success I've had, or will have in life, is due in great part to my family.

It would be a crime not to thank God for my friends, past and present. *There is no greater gift in life than knowing fabulous people, and I happen to know many. I'm grateful for having been a part of their lives.* There's been a great support system that has got me as far as I have come. Without them, where I would be? I have not gotten to where I am today by myself! A lot of time, energy, and money has been invested in me. As they say, it takes a village. Some of these wonderful people have passed away, and I feel a great void inside me. Not only have I lost them, but the whole world misses them for all their wonderful qualities that are no longer available. There are some I have not mentioned here, but that does not mean they were treasured any less.

Count your blessings. Despite this disorder, I must count my blessings. It has been very tough dealing with multiple bizarre symptoms at one time, but I am truly thankful for the abilities I still have and the abilities that have come back to some degree. Although everyone with dystonia has the same basic symptoms—repetitive, involuntary movements—the severity of the symptoms and the regions of the body that are affected are unique to every sufferer. I feel I may have one of the more severe strains, because no treatment has ever had any tangible or lasting effect. Nothing that helps or offers relief is ever planned and can seldom be duplicated. It just happens. Where would I be had they not hit that blood vessel during brain surgery? I was spared a more hellish existence by that stroke. It was a stroke of luck! But no matter how bad things have gotten for me, I know there is always someone worse off than I am!

Had I been given the chance to say *no* to this disorder, of course I would have. But the experiences I've had and the people I've met are unique unto themselves. I've seen the human condition up close and it has been compelling. Without dystonia, I wouldn't have the same perspective of life. Whether that perspective would be better or worse I'll never know for sure.

I'm also grateful for technology. If it weren't for technology, I doubt this book would ever have come to being. With the way I type (I can use one finger on my left hand) and the mistakes I make, I would not have had the energy or patience the writing process demands with a normal and nearly out-dated typewriter. I would have never guessed it would take well over five years to write it, but there were times I had to walk away and leave it for a while. I was busy with other things, and my rebellious body was not up to doing them and writing all at once. But my thoughts were always with it. I never let myself forget most of the experiences you have read about in this book. (Mom's notes filled in the memory gaps.) I never thought those experiences would make it out of my head and onto paper. I didn't know why I carried these memories around. Why couldn't I let them go? I thought they were significant only to me!

Technology can either help or hinder, but it makes a disabled person's life much easier. If I had been born in a time period before surgery, medications, and wheelchairs—especially electric ones—I wouldn't have had any positive quality of life to speak about!

I believe that we are all, at some point in our lives, sent on an unexpected detour —something we have no control over that we just have to accept and deal with. What form it will take we don't know, but it will test our strength. When this happens, do not put your life on hold, and do not be devastated by challenge and change. Tap into the resources that work for you to help you find your own strength. It takes time, but it's worth it.

My faith and relationship with God is very strong, but has been shaky at times. I've had many occasions where God has made his presence very real, and I know he will always be there—even if it's not evident at the time! I don't think that I have ever blamed God for my condition, but I have some unanswered questions!

Learn from the past, but live in the present. Most of my experiences in life, some traumatic and some rare, were undesirable at the time but taught me invaluable lessons. For the most part I would not change too much, but I would like to do a few of my teenage years over again to skip the self-esteem issues, the naivety, the high volume of medication, and the daydreaming from all happening at once. I wish I had the confidence in myself then that I have now! You cannot make someone believe they can do something until they're ready and convinced that it is possible. I wish a person could. That was my case.

I am not the person to come to if you're seeking advice or secrets about living successfully with dystonia, for I don't have all the answers, even for myself. But I have found that stretching my muscles as much and as often as I feel comfortable doing helps me stay flexible. The key is to find a balance between activity and down time! Sometimes I have to give up something I value very much in order to achieve another goal.

I used to think that physical therapy was a terrible waste of time because it required me to do stretches and get into "proper positions" I could not hold. Walking in parallel bars and balance testing was so awkward. I wish I would have caught on to the benefits of therapy earlier, but I could barely cope with the sudden, aggressive symptoms that were changing my life. It was just so difficult, frustrating, and overwhelming.

In my early twenties, my activity was not as hectic as the years before, and I started to take exercise more seriously. I gained better endurance so I could slowly start to do some things that I couldn't do before and actually enjoy doing them. Generally speaking, able bodies are taught how to clean, cook, and do other tasks that I obviously couldn't do in my younger years, so I find learning all kinds of new things quite liberating!

For the past few years I have been seeing a physical therapist at least twice a year which is wonderful, because I went for many years without seeing one. Stretching is a total must. It is vital to be as flexible as possible. I still work out to keep up my energy and endurance level too. I don't exercise with as much intensity as I once did, partly because if I'm having a very spastic day I'm probably doing more harm than good and my muscles aren't quite as cooperative as they were at the start. But I do like, and realize the need for, exercise.

Recently I discovered that it is best to do stretches right before I lie down to sleep. Easing any soreness or stiffness is especially important at that time. It can be easier to fall asleep when my muscles are loose and relaxed. If after a period of inactivity while sleeping or on the couch, I feel stiff, then moving around usually makes that feeling go away. It is ironic that moving sometimes help solve that problem because moving *is* my problem! I do make the best of it, and I find it impossible to leave anything on a bad note when I know that my life has not all been bad! It has never been easy but I am blessed with better days! My life has been, and can continue to be very rich and fulfilling at times. That is my focus.

It is hard to fathom that this disease has been with me for so many years and that it will be with me for the rest of my life unless, of course, they do find a cure or an effective treatment.

When I asked my world-renowned pediatric neurologist, Dr. Gauk (retired), whom I still keep in touch with, if he believes dystonia will be cured in my lifetime he responded, "If you knew how many diseases have been cured since I was in medical school fifty years ago... I wouldn't be surprised."

What Are the
Many Forms of Dystonia?

Focal Dystonias

Focal dystonias are adult-onset forms that affects a specific area of the body. Most focal dystonias are primary (meaning that it is the only neurological symptom and presumed to have a genetic component), though secondary cases are documented. Focal dystonia may affect muscles of the eyes, mouth, vocal cords, neck, hands, and feet. Types of focal dystonia include:

- Blepharospasm—Affects the eyes
- Cervical dystonia (spasmodic torticollis)—Affects neck and shoulders
- Oromandibular dystonia (cranial dystonia)—Affects face, mouth, and/or jaw
- Laryngeal dystonia (spasmodic dysphonia)—Affects the vocal cords
- Hand dystonia (writer's cramp)—Affects the hands and forearm

Musicians' Dystonias

Professional musicians are susceptible to a variety of specific occupational injuries. One disorder to which musicians are susceptible is task-specific focal dystonia.

Hand dystonia and embouchure dystonia (which affects the mouth, cheeks, jaw, and tongue) are the types of dystonia most often diagnosed in musicians. Playing the instrument triggers the muscle spasms. The spasms are not usually present at rest.

Musicians may perceive the early symptoms of dystonia as the result of faulty technique or lack of sufficient preparation. By definition, musicians' dystonia is almost always focal and does not spread to affect additional parts of the body.

Early-onset Generalized Dystonia

Early-onset generalized dystonia is characterized by the twisting of the limbs, specifically the foot and leg or hand and arm. The spasms may spread to involve twisting contractions of other parts of the body.

Early onset dystonia can be broadly divided into two major categories: DYT1 early onset generalized dystonia and non-DYT1 early onset dystonia. The distinction is that DYT1 generalized dystonia is known to be caused by a specific mutation in the DYT1 gene. However, not all primary generalized dystonias that begin in childhood are caused by this specific mutation in this gene. These forms are simply referred to as non-DYT1 generalized dystonia.

DYT1 dystonia is primary. Non-DYT1 dystonia may be primary or secondary.

Terms used to describe DYT1 generalized dystonia include: Oppenheim's dystonia, primary torsion dystonia, early onset dystonia, childhood onset dystonia, idiopathic torsion dystonia. Lesser-used terms include: dystonia musculum deformans

Terms used to describe non-DYT1 generalized dystonia include: Primary torsion dystonia, early onset dystonia, childhood onset dystonia, idiopathic torsion dystonia. Lesser-used terms include: dystonia musculorum deformans

Historically, early-onset generalized dystonia has also been referred to as idiopathic torsion dystonia and dystonia musculorum deformans.

Dopa-responsive dystonia

Dopa-responsive dystonia (DRD) is a broad term used to describe forms of dystonia that respond to a medication called levodopa, which is a synthetic form of a brain chemical called dopamine. This group includes heredity forms that are characterized by progressive difficulty walking. Its symptoms may be similar to those of early onset generalized dystonia.

Terms used to describe dopa-responsive dystonia include: DRD, Segawa's dystonia, Segawa's disease, DYT5 dystonia

Myoclonic dystonia

Myoclonic dystonia, a genetic form of dystonia, is characterized by rapid jerking movements alone or in combination with the sustained muscular contractions and postures of dystonia.

Terms used to describe myoclonic dystonia include: myoclonus dystonia, inherited myoclonus-dystonia syndrome, DYT11 dystonia

Note: Some researchers believe myoclonic dystonia is a variation of hereditary essential myoclonus.

Paroxysmal dystonia and dyskinesias

Paroxysmal dyskinesias (PD) are episodic movement disorders in which abnormal movements are present only during attacks. The term paroxysmal indicates that symptoms are noticeable only at certain times. The term dyskinesia broadly refers to movements of the body that are involuntary. Between attacks most people are generally neurologically normal, and there is no loss of consciousness during the attacks.

Rapid-onset dystonia-parkinsonism

Rapid-onset dystonia Parkinsonism (RDP), a hereditary form of dystonia, is characterized by the abrupt onset of slowness of movement (parkinsonism) and dystonic symptoms.

Terms used to describe rapid-onset dystonia-parkinsonism include: DRP, DYT12 dystonia

X-linked Dystonia-parkinsonism

X-linked dystonia-parkinsonism (XDP) is a genetic form of dystonia found almost entirely among males of Filipino descent.

Terms used to describe X-linked dystonia-parkinsonism include: XDP, Lubag

Secondary Dystonias

The various forms of dystonia can be divided into two broad groups: primary dystonias and secondary dystonias. Primary dystonias are genetic (or believed to be genetic) in origin, whereas secondary dystonias result from apparent outside factors and can be attributed to a specific cause such as exposure to certain medications, trauma, toxins, infections, or stroke.

Secondary dystonia is dystonia that develops mainly as the result of environmental factors that provide insult to the brain. Spinal cord, head, and peripheral injury are also recognized contributors to dystonia. Other examples of secondary dystonias include levodopa-induced dystonia in the treatment of parkinsonism; acute and tardive dystonia due to specific drugs such as dopamine receptor blocking agents; and dystonias associated with cerebral palsy, cerebral hypoxia, cerebrovascular disease, cerebral infections and postinfectious states, stroke, encephalitis, brain tumor, and toxins such as manganese, cyanide, and 3-nitroproprionic acid.

Many secondary dystonias are dystonias associated with approximately 50 neurological and metabolic diseases. Many of these diseases are genetic. This category includes diseases such as corticobasal degeneration, pantothenate kinase deficiency (aka Hallorvorden-Spatz), Huntington's disease, Wilson's disease, Leigh's disease, and juvenile parkinsonism.

A number of secondary dystonias do not present as pure dystonia, but with a mixture of other neurologic features, such as parkinsonian features like slowness of movement (bradykinesia) and rigidity.

Printed from the DMRFC website, with permission.

A Twisted Fate

For more information about dystonia,
- visit the DMFRC website at <u>www.dystoniacanada.org</u>
- call them toll free at 800-361-8061 for service in English or 800-787-1015 for service in French.
- In the U.S.A. visit <u>www.dystonia-foundation.org</u> or call toll free at 800-377-3978

       Donations are always welcome!

CPSIA information can be obtained at www.ICGtesting.com
Printed in the USA
LVOW08s0630280415

436375LV00001B/12/P